Nutrition in Critical Care

Nutrition in Critical Care

Edited by

Peter Faber, MD, PhD, FRCA, FFICM

Consultant Cardio-Thoracic Anaesthetist,
Department of Cardiac Anaesthesia,
Aberdeen Royal Infirmary, Aberdeen, UK

Mario Siervo, MD, MSc, PhD, RPHN

Lecturer in Nutrition and Ageing,
Human Nutrition Research Centre,
Institute for Ageing and Health,
Newcastle University, Newcastle upon Tyne, UK

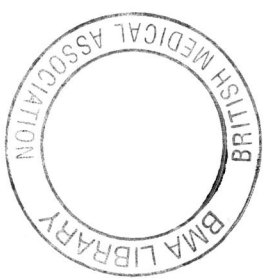

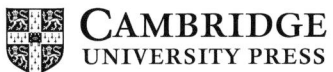

CAMBRIDGE
UNIVERSITY PRESS

CAMBRIDGE
UNIVERSITY PRESS

University Printing House, Cambridge CB2 8BS, United Kingdom

Published in the United States of America by Cambridge University Press, New York

Cambridge University Press is part of the University of Cambridge.

It furthers the University's mission by disseminating knowledge in the pursuit of
education, learning, and research at the highest international levels of excellence.

www.cambridge.org
Information on this title: www.cambridge.org/9781107669017

© Cambridge University Press 2014

First published 2014

Printed and bound in the United Kingdom by Bell and Bain Ltd

A catalog record for this publication is available from the British Library

Library of Congress Cataloging in Publication data
Nutrition in critical care (Faber)
Nutrition in critical care / edited by Peter Faber, Mario Siervo.
    p. ; cm.
Includes bibliographical references and index.
ISBN 978-1-107-66901-7 (paperback)
I. Faber, Peter, 1969– editor of compilation.   II. Siervo, Mario, editor of
compilation.   III. Title.
[DNLM: 1. Nutritional Support.   2. Critical Care. WB 410]
RM217
615.8′54–dc23

                                                        2013036992

ISBN 978-1-107-66901-7 Paperback

Contents

List of contributors

BJARNE F. ALSBJOERN, MD, DMSCI
Consultant Surgeon, Director of Burns Unit, Copenhagen University Hospital, Copenhagen East, Denmark

CAROLINE M. APOVIAN, MD
Professor of Medicine, Boston University School of Medicine, Nutrition and Weight Management Center, Boston, MA, USA

DANNY COLLINS
Department of Anaesthesia, Papworth Hospital, Papworth Everard, Cambridge, UK

ROLAND N. DICKERSON, PHARMD, BCNSP, FACN, FCCP, FASHP, FCCM
Professor of Clinical Pharmacy, University of Tennessee Health Science Center, and Clinical Coordinator and Clinical Pharmacist, Nutrition Support Service, Regional Medical Center at Memphis, Memphis, TN, USA

TIMOTHY EDEN
Great Western Hospitals NHS Foundation Trust, Swindon;
Medical Research Council Human Nutrition Research Unit, Cambridge;
and The Need for Nutrition Education Programme, c/o British Dietetic Association, Birmingham, UK

PETER FABER, MD, PHD, FRCA, FFICM
Consultant Cardio-Thoracic Anaesthetist, Department of Cardiac Anaesthesia, Aberdeen Royal Infirmary, Aberdeen, UK

ANDREW J. FERGUSON
Consultant in Anaesthesia and Intensive Care Medicine, Craigavon Area Hospital, Northern Ireland, UK

DAVID C. FRANKENFIELD, MS, RD
Chief Clinical Dietitian, Department of Clinical Nutrition, Penn State Milton S. Hershey Medical Center, Hershey, PA, USA

DYMPNA GALLAGHER, EDD
Associate Professor of Nutritional Medicine, Department of Medicine and Institute of Human Nutrition, Columbia University;
Director, Body Composition Unit, New York Obesity and Nutrition Research Center, St. Luke's-Roosevelt Hospital, New York, NY, USA

MARIA GABRIELLA GENTILE
Director, Eating Disorders Unit, Niguarda Hospital, Milan, Italy

WILSON I. GONSALVES, MD
Department of Oncology, Mayo Clinic, Rochester, MN, USA

ANDREW M. HETREED, MBBS, BSC, FRCA
Specialist Registrar in Anaesthetics and Intensive Care, Addenbrooke's Hospital, Cambridge, UK

MICHAEL H. HOOPER
Department of Medicine, Division of Pulmonary and Critical Care Medicine, Eastern Virginia Medical School, Norfolk, VA, USA

JAN O. JANSEN
Consultant in General Surgery and Intensive Care Medicine, Aberdeen Royal Infirmary, Aberdeen, UK

AMINAH JATOI, MD
Department of Oncology, Mayo Clinic, Rochester, MN, USA

YING JI, MD
Research Fellow, New York Obesity and Nutrition Research Center, St. Luke's-Roosevelt Hospital, New York, NY, USA

ILYA KAGAN
Department of Intensive Care, Beilinson Hospital, Rabin Medical Center, Sackler School of Medicine, Tel Aviv University, Tel Aviv, Israel

ANDREW J. KERWIN, MD
Associate Professor of Surgery, Division Chief, Acute Care Surgery, Department of Surgery, University of Florida College of Medicine, Jacksonville; and Trauma Medical Director, Shands Jacksonville Medical Center, Jacksonville, FL, USA

DONG WOOK KIM, MD
Instructor of Medicine, Boston University School of Medicine, Nutrition and Weight Management Center, Boston, MA, USA

ANDREW A. KLEIN
Department of Anaesthesia, Papworth Hospital, Papworth Everard, Cambridge, UK

ALISTAIR LEE, FRCA
Consultant in Transplant Anaesthesia and Critical Care, Department of Anaesthesia, Critical Care & Pain Medicine, Royal Infirmary of Edinburgh, Edinburgh, UK

SHAUL LEV
Department of Intensive Care, Beilinson Hospital, Rabin Medical Center, Sackler School of Medicine, Tel Aviv University, Tel Aviv, Israel

PETER K. LINDEN, MD
Professor of Medicine and Critical Care Medicine, Temple University School of Medicine, Allegheny General Hospital, Pittsburgh, PA, USA

PAUL E. MARIK
Department of Medicine, Division of Pulmonary and Critical Care Medicine, Eastern Virginia Medical School, Norfolk, VA, USA

ROBERT MARTINDALE, MD, PHD, FACS
Chief, General Surgery Division, Oregon Health Sciences University, Portland, OR, USA

PETER McCANNY
Department of Anaesthesia and Intensive Care, Saint James Hospital, Dublin, Ireland

PAOLO MERLANI
Intensive Care Unit, Geneva University Hospital and University of Geneva, Geneva, Switzerland

SHAY NANTHAKUMARAN
Consultant Surgeon, Aberdeen Royal Infirmary, Aberdeen, UK

MICHAEL S. NUSSBAUM, MD
Professor and Chair, Department of Surgery, University of Florida College of Medicine, Jacksonville, and Surgeon-in-Chief, Shands Jacksonville Medical Center, Jacksonville, FL, USA

ANDREAS PERREN
Intensive Care Unit, Ospedale Regionale Bellinzona e Valli, Bellinzona, Switzerland

CARLA PRADO
Department of Nutrition, Food and Exercise Sciences, College of Human Sciences, The Florida State University, Tallahassee, FL, USA

JEAN-CHARLES PREISER, MD, PHD
Department of Intensive Care, Erasme University Hospital, Brussels, Belgium

MINHA RAJPUT-RAY
Cambridge University Hospitals NHS Foundation Trust, Cambridge; Medical Research Council Human Nutrition Research Unit, Cambridge; and The Need for Nutrition Education Programme, c/o British Dietetic Association, Birmingham, UK

SUMANTRA RAY
Cambridge University Hospitals NHS Foundation Trust, Cambridge; Medical Research Council Human Nutrition Research Unit, Cambridge; and The Need for Nutrition Education Programme, c/o British Dietetic Association, Birmingham, UK

NILS SIEGENTHALER
Intensive Care Unit, Geneva University Hospital and University of Geneva, Geneva, Switzerland

MARIO SIERVO, MD, MSC, PHD, RPHN
Lecturer in Nutrition and Ageing, Human Nutrition Research Centre, Institute for Ageing and Health, Newcastle University, Newcastle upon Tyne, UK

JONATHAN A. SILVERSIDES
Clinical Fellow in Critical Care Medicine, Toronto General Hospital, Toronto, Canada

PIERRE SINGER
Department of Intensive Care, Beilinson Hospital, Rabin Medical Center, Sackler School of Medicine, Tel Aviv University, Tel Aviv, Israel

JOHN A. TAYEK, MD, FACP, FACN
Professor of Medicine – In Residence, David Geffen School of Medicine, Harbor-UCLA Medical Center, Torrance, CA, USA

EUAN THOMSON, MRCP, FRCA
Consultant Anaesthetist, Department of Anaesthesia, Critical Care & Pain Medicine, Royal Infirmary of Edinburgh, Edinburgh, UK

KRISTA L. TURNER, MD, FACS
Assistant Professor, Department of Surgery, The Methodist Hospital, Weill Cornell Medical College, Houston, TX, USA

MALISSA WARREN, RD, CNSC
Portland VA Medical Center, Portland, OR, USA

STEPHEN T. WEBB
Consultant in Cardiothoracic Anaesthesia and Intensive Care Medicine, Papworth Hospital, Papworth Everard, Cambridge, UK

PATRICIA WIESEN, MD
Department of General Intensive Care, University Hospital Center of Liege, Liege, Belgium

Preface

Nutritional sciences have rapidly expanded within the last few decades with an increasing amount of studies available to guide best evidence practice. Nutrition and the effects of too little, too much, and not the right composition are publicly discussed almost daily amongst the press and politicians. Everybody appears to have an opinion when it comes to the benefits and damages to human health by either the right or wrong diet. Unfortunately, many of these views are carried over into professional healthcare in hospitals where the nutritional support of patients often does not receive adequate attention. Technological and medicinal development in patient care may often result in the nutritional needs of patients being pushed down the list of priorities. Additionally, a lack of personal scientific knowledge of nutrition may result in many clinicians and healthcare workers steering clear of engaging with the nutritional requirements of patients and the benefits optimal diets offer to patient care. No more so is this true than within the critical care environment. Frequently, nutritional assessment and management is not comprehensively integrated into overall patient care. Fortunately, due to the increasing public interest in health and nutrition many clinicians are now starting to engage with nutritional sciences as a tool to improve patient care and prognosis.

The editors of this book have assembled contributions from internationally recognized authors to assist healthcare professionals working within the critical care environment in implementing current best evidence in nutritional support of patients. With this book, it is the hope of the editors not only to provide nutritional support guidelines for the various group of patients admitted to the Critical Care Unit, but also to allow a basic scientific knowledge aiding clinical discussions and decisions. This book should prove useful to those studying nutrition in critical care, but it may also provide an accessible guide for the resident to assist with the nutritional assessment of patients and therapeutic strategies. The book is aimed at doctors, nurses, dieticians, and practitioners working within the critical care environment.

The editors would like to thank all the contributing authors. Without their time and dedication this book would not have happened. We would also like to thank Cambridge University Press, and especially Joanna Chamberlin and Nisha Doshi, for accepting this project and assisting us in getting it completed.

1

Nutritional physiology of the critically ill patient

David C. Frankenfield

Introduction

Nutritional physiology refers to the role of food and nutrition in the function of the body. In the critically ill patient there are numerous points at which nutrition affects function, since all fuels, tissues, and mediators ultimately arise from the food consumed by the individual. There are now evidence-based guidelines for the provision of nutrition support in the critically ill patient. Several actions related to feeding improve outcomes such as infection rate, days on mechanical ventilation, days in the critical care unit, and mortality. These actions include the provision of early enteral nutrition, use of tube feedings supplemented with n-3 fatty acids and antioxidants, and reaching minimum targets for energy and protein intake. The minimum target range is an area of debate currently.

This chapter will focus on energy balance, protein and nitrogen balance, and the macronutrient requirements of critically ill patients compared to normal. The potential role of nutrients to modulate inflammatory injury in the critically ill patient will also be examined.

Energy

All functions of the body require energy. Ultimately all energy used by the body is consumed in the diet. Some is used immediately and some is converted to glycogen or body tissue to be used later. In healthy people ingested fuel is used when available and suppresses the use of stored fuel. Stored fuel is mobilized post-prandially as the ingested fuel is consumed. In critically ill patients this priority is altered, with ongoing use of stored fuel, especially protein, even if dietary fuel is available.

Nutrition in Critical Care, ed. Peter Faber and Mario Siervo. Published by Cambridge University Press. © Cambridge University Press 2014.

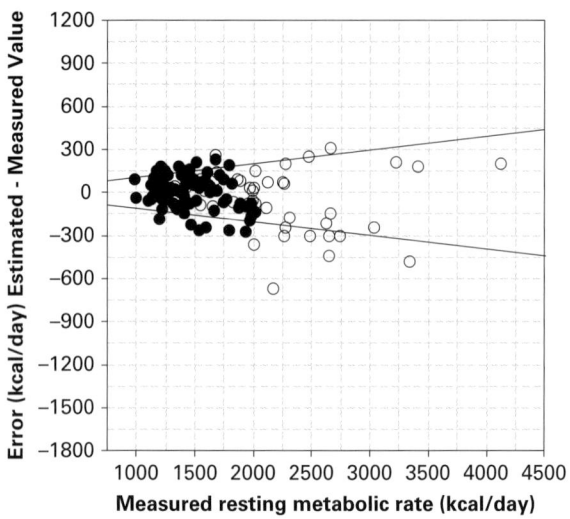

Figure 1.1 Errors in predicting resting metabolic rate using the Mifflin–St. Jeor equation in healthy individuals. Closed circles are patients with body mass index < 30 kg/m^2 and open circles are patients with body mass index ≥ 30 kg/m^2. Within the central band are predictions falling within 10% of measured. Negative values are underestimates and positive values are overestimates. The accuracy rate of the equation in non-obese individuals was 82% compared to 70% in obese people.

In healthy people resting metabolic rate is determined by energy expenditure in the visceral organs. Through relationships among organ mass, fat-free mass, and body weight, resting metabolic rate is predictable from body weight, height, age, and sex. The Mifflin–St. Jeor equation, for example, can predict resting metabolic rate accurately in healthy people about 75% of the time (Figure 1.1). These equations take the following form:

- Resting metabolic rate (men) (kcal/day) = Wt in kg(10) + Ht in cm(6.25) – Age in yrs(5) +5
- Resting metabolic rate (women) (kcal/day) = Wt in kg(10) + Ht in cm(6.25) – Age in yrs(5) – 161.

In critically ill patients, the relationship between body size and resting metabolic rate is still present. However, the utilization rate of fuel is accelerated in the critically ill patient. The hormonal milieu is characterized by a decrease in the ratio of insulin to glucagon, increased catecholamine levels, and insulin resistance. A host of cytokine and eicosanoid mediators also are present, creating an inflammatory response. Under the influence of these mediators the critically ill body increases its rate of gluconeogenesis, proteolysis, acute phase protein production, lipolysis, and oxygen consumption. Energy expenditure is increased on average by about 25%, but there is wide variability, from 25% below expected

Table 1.1 Elevation in resting metabolic rate in critical care patients (as a percentage of predicted healthy resting metabolic rate as estimated by the Mifflin–St. Jeor equation)

		All			Febrile		Afebrile	
Group	N	Mean ± SD	Range	Percent febrile in previous 24 hours	Mean ± SD	Range	Mean ± SD	Range
Trauma	52	1.30 ± 0.18	0.99–2.1	69	1.32 ± 0.19	1.09–2.14	1.24 ± 0.17	0.99–1.77
Surgical	65	1.22 ± 0.17	0.92–1.8	46	1.26 ± 0.16	0.97–1.60	1.19 ± 0.18	0.92–1.83
Medical	85	1.21 ± 0.20	0.75–1.8	38	1.31 ± 0.20	0.93–1.76	1.15 ± 0.17	0.75–1.51
Total	202	1.23 ± 0.19	0.75–2.1	49	1.30 ± 0.18	0.93–2.14	1.18 ± 0.17	0.75–1.83

Data from Frankenfield DC, Schubert A, Alam S, Cooney RN. Validation study of predictive equations for resting metabolic rate in critically ill patients. JPEN J Parenter Ent Nutr 2009;33:27–36.

healthy metabolic rate to more than two times elevation above expected healthy value (Table 1.1).

The increase is not related to illness severity as measured by APACHE (Acute Physiology and Chronic Health Evaluation) score, or by type of illness/injury. However, body temperature does discriminate the degree of hypermetabolism. The respiratory effort, measured as minute ventilation, also increases as more fuel consumption results in more carbon dioxide production that must be removed by the lungs. These physiological changes can be exploited to predict the increase in energy expenditure. The Penn State equations use the Mifflin–St. Jeor equation to capture the association between resting metabolic rate and body size, and then use body temperature and minute ventilation to account for the metabolic effects of inflammatory response:

- Resting metabolic rate (kcal/day) = Mifflin(0.96) + Tmax(167) + Ve(31) – 6212
- Resting metabolic rate (kcal/day) = Mifflin(0.74) + Tmax(85) + Ve(64) – 3085

where Mifflin is Mifflin–St. Jeor equation, Tmax is maximum body temperature in the previous 24 hours (centigrade), and Ve is minute ventilation (L/min).

Using this equation, resting metabolic rate can be predicted accurately about 75% of the time (Figure 1.2).

Over time, indirect calorimetry measurements must be repeated every 3 to 4 days to be more accurate than daily recalculation of metabolic rate using the Penn State equation (Figure 1.3). Other common prediction methods such as the Harris–Benedict equation or the rule of thumb from the American College of Chest Physicians (25 kcal/kg body weight) are accurate at best 50% of the time, and in the case of the ACCP (American College of Chest Physicians) standard there is proportional bias (increasing underestimation as measured metabolic rate increases).

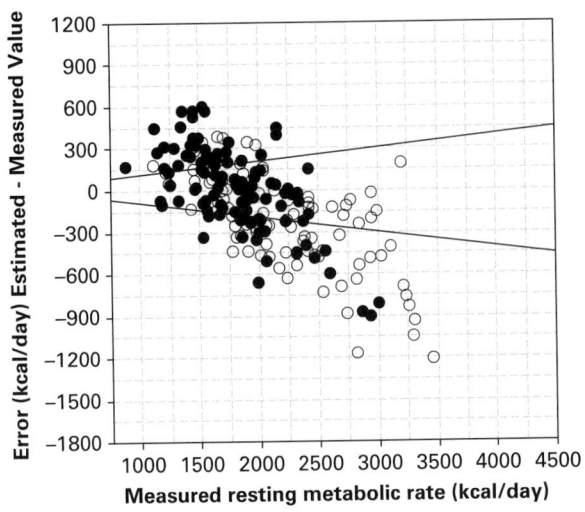

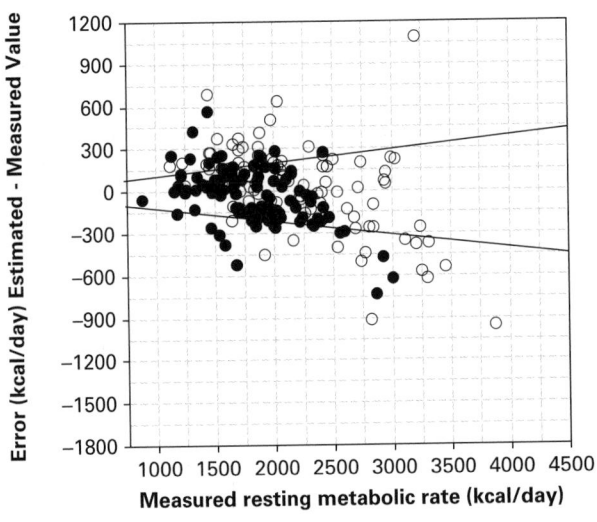

Figure 1.2 Errors in predicting resting metabolic rate using the ACCP standard of 25 kcal/kg body weight (top) and the Penn State equation (bottom). Closed circles are patients with body mass index < 30 kg/m^2 and open circles are patients with body mass index ≥ 30 kg/m^2. Within the central band are predictions falling within 10% of measured. Negative values are underestimates and positive values are overestimates. For the ACCP standard, estimates were accurate 52% of the time vs 67% for the Penn State equation. With a modification to the equation for patients 60 years or older with body mass index 30 kg/m^2 or higher, the overall accuracy of the Penn State equation increases to 73%.

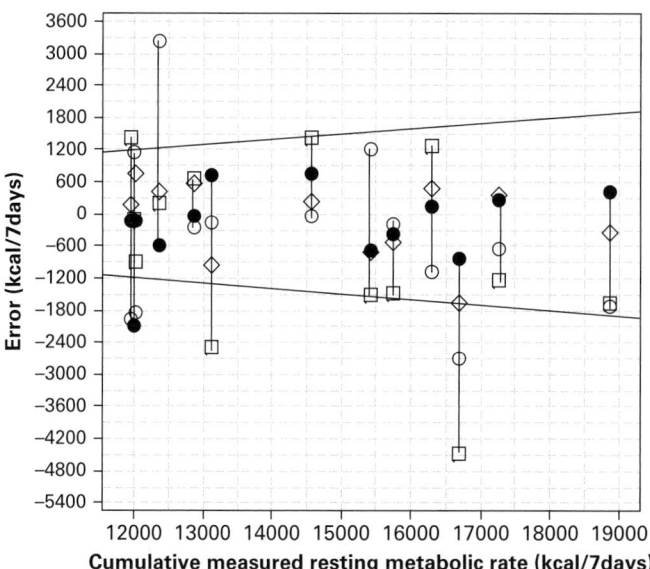

Figure 1.3 Cumulative errors in predicting resting metabolic rate in mechanically ventilated critically ill patients using the Penn State equation (closed circles), ACCP standard of 25 kcal/kg (open circles), a 7-day estimate extrapolated from a single measurement (open squares), and a 7-day estimate extrapolated from two measures on day 1 and day 4 (open diamonds). The vertical lines connect the four estimates for a single patient. Total number of patients studied was 13.

Protein

There is general agreement that protein needs are elevated in the critically ill patient, but there is little agreement as to the exact requirement. The critically ill patient experiences an increase in muscle proteolysis that is resistant to the usual attenuating effect of feeding. Nitrogen and muscle loss are moderately correlated with the degree of hypermetabolism (R^2 0.25 and 0.37 respectively). Proteolysis in critically ill patients is thought to occur in order to mobilize amino acids from muscle to be used in the viscera for gluconeogenesis, acute phase protein synthesis, RNA, and ATP. The availability of glutamine to the viscera may play an extraordinary role in this movement of amino acids from the periphery to the central tissues of the body, serving as a major fuel and cell component in the cells of the immune system and gastrointestinal tract, an antioxidant (glutathione), and a component of acid–base balance in the kidney.

Thus the critically ill patient is at once experiencing increased catabolism (muscle) and increased synthesis (viscera), but the net effect is a catabolic state resistant to feeding. Nutrition support is capable of stimulating the synthetic component but cannot eliminate the catabolic component.

Table 1.2 Nitrogen utilization at different levels of energy balance in critically ill patients

Parameter	Burge		Dickerson	Frankenfield		
	Hypocaloric	Eucaloric	Hypocaloric	Hypocaloric	Eucaloric	Hypercaloric
Percentage of kilo calories fed	73	113	63	75	105	124
Nitrogen intake (g/d)	18	21	21	19	19	20
Nitrogen output (g/d)	8	11	15	27	25	27
Balance (g/d)	+1	+3	+2	−8	−8	−8
Catabolic rate (g/d)	64	85	–	90	105	95

Data compiled from Dickerson RN, Rosato EF, Mullen JL. Net protein anabolism with hypocaloric parenteral nutrition in obese stressed patients. Am J Clin Nutr 1986;44:747–755; Burge JC, Goon A, Choban PS, Flancbaum L. Efficacy of hypocaloric total parenteral nutrition in hospitalized obese patients: a prospective, double-blind randomized trial. J Parenter Enteral Nutr 1994;18:203–207; Frankenfield DC, Smith JS, Cooney RN. Accelerated nitrogen loss after traumatic injury is not attenuated by achievement of energy balance. J Parenter Enteral Nutr 1997;21:324–329.

Another unique aspect of protein metabolism in the critically ill patient is its relationship with energy intake. In healthy people nitrogen balance can only be achieved when energy balance is also achieved and the protein intake is adequate. At a fixed but inadequate protein intake, nitrogen balance will improve as more total energy is fed but a plateau in nitrogen balance will occur before nitrogen equilibrium. At a fixed and inadequate energy intake, nitrogen balance will improve as more protein is fed but again a plateau in nitrogen balance will occur before equilibrium is achieved (unless so much protein is given that the requirement for total energy is satisfied). In critically ill patients, there are studies in which nitrogen balance has been demonstrated to be independent of energy balance (Table 1.2).

Research on this topic has focused either exclusively on obese patients or included non-obese and obese patients. Obese patients were not as catabolic as the non-obese patients (consisting of blunt trauma patients studied in the first week after injury). The nitrogen losses in obese patients were lower than in non-obese patients, and thus nitrogen balance was positive. Non-obese patients reached similar nitrogen intake to the two studies on obese patients but had much higher nitrogen losses and thus did not achieve nitrogen balance. However, over a wider range of energy intake, nitrogen balance was not more negative in underfed than in overfed patients. Muscle catabolic rate was likewise found to be independent of energy intake, though it must be made clear that none of the patients studied were completely unfed during the study and all received protein. Studies of catabolic rate in which only low concentration dextrose (5%) was given show a higher catabolic rate than demonstrated in studies of fed patients.

Balance studies

Bartlett published perhaps the first study of the effect of negative energy balance on outcomes in the critical care unit. In an observational study of 57 critical care patients whose resting metabolic rate was measured once or twice each day of their intensive care unit stay, mortality rate was 27% in 15 patients achieving positive energy balance, 39% in 28 patients with an energy balance of 0 to −10 000 kcal, and 86% in 14 patients with an energy deficit greater than 10 000 kcal. Subsequent observational studies have disputed this finding, showing detrimental outcome associated with more aggressive provision of energy. Most recently, however, several studies indicate an outcome advantage to meeting the energy and protein demand of critically ill patients via nutrition support.

One prospective randomized clinical trial has been conducted to examine the question of energy balance in critically ill patients. The study used indirect calorimetry to monitor actual energy expenditure in 112 critically ill patients. One group was assigned a study coordinator to adjust feeding rates to compensate for interruptions so that energy intake matched (actually exceeded) the measured energy expenditure (cumulative balance +2008 ± 2177 kcal over 14 days) while the other group was randomized to standard care in which the feeding interruptions common in critical care were not compensated for by rate adjustment, resulting in negative energy balance of −3550 ± 4591 kcal over 14 days. Length of stay in the critical care unit was significantly longer in the group in positive energy balance (16 vs 11 days) as were days on mechanical ventilation (17 vs 12 days), but overall hospital mortality rate was reduced from 48% to 29%. It should be noted that the positive energy balance group also received a higher protein intake than the negative energy balance group. Besides the prospective randomized nature of design of this study, another unique aspect was the extension of the examination of outcomes of critical care interventions in the post-critical care environment.

In a study of 50 septic patients requiring continuous renal replacement therapy it was found that positive nitrogen balance conferred a survival advantage (a 21% increase in survival probability was noted for a 1 g/day increase in nitrogen balance). Increasing protein intake was associated with an improvement in nitrogen balance, but not directly with an improvement in survival. This may be because some septic patients are less able to utilize the dietary protein than others. Those who can utilize the protein more efficiently are more likely to achieve positive nitrogen balance, and the data indicate that this ability results in a survival advantage. Therefore it was recommended a protein intake > 2.0 g/kg body weight (ideally 2.5 g/kg body weight).

A larger (n=886) study of general critical care patients found that achieving protein and energy intake goals reduced the 28-day and overall hospital mortality risk. The reduction in risk was even more pronounced when the data were controlled for age, body mass index, admitting diagnosis, APACHE score, hyperglycemia index, and time to reach target intake. Notably, energy balance alone did not reduce the mortality risk.

Water

In healthy people, water intake should balance losses both sensible and insensible. A general rule is 30 mL/kg body weight. In the critically ill patient the same is often but not always true, and fluid needs can change as the illness evolves. Early on in the illness and during septic shock while the vascular system is dilated, the need for water and volume are increased. If acute renal failure has occurred, then water requirements can be decreased. On the other hand water loss during continuous renal replacement therapy can be many liters per day and require extra replacement. Chronic illness such as congestive heart failure may continue to dictate fluid restriction even during a period of critical illness. High water loss through the gastrointestinal tract as gastric drainage or diarrhea, or high fluid loss through surgical drains will increase the need for fluid replacement. It is important to realize that water needs often need to be met not simply with water but with crystalloid or colloidal fluids. Remove these from the dietary fluid needs of the patient, and further subtracting the obligatory fluid intake from medications, and the water content of a nutrition support regimen may actually need to be restricted even though the patient's overall requirement for fluid is increased.

Nutrition and inflammation

Injury and infection elicit inflammatory responses from the host that help create the conditions to resolve the insult and return the body to a state of homeostasis. This is accomplished through orchestration of anti-inflammatory and pro-inflammatory processes. However, if multiple insults occur, or if the response to a single insult is severe, the inflammatory response becomes dysregulated and maladaptive, leading to hemodynamic and other organ and metabolic dysfunction, and ultimately to increased morbidity and mortality. Many of the mediators of inflammation are produced from dietary components, especially fatty acids. A change in diet can be rapidly detected in the fatty acid composition of cell membranes and enteral feeding formulas containing n-3 fatty acids have been shown to improve outcomes in patients with inflammatory lung disease and sepsis. Specifically, a prospective randomized clinical trial has been conducted on critically ill patients with sepsis or septic shock. All of the patients also met criteria for acute respiratory distress syndrome. The patients were randomized to one of two high-fat diets. The control diet was based on canola oil while the treatment diet contained canola, borage, and fish oil, nearly doubling the ratio of n-3:n-6 from 1:3.8 to 1:1.85. Starting at the fourth day of the study, PaO_2/FIO_2 ratio fell in the study group compared to the control as a result of increased PaO_2 as well as decreased FIO_2. Accompanying this improvement in oxygenation was a fall in positive end-expiratory pressure (PEEP) and minute ventilation. In the 28-day study period the treatment group had more ventilator-free days (13 vs 6) and more ICU-free days (11 vs 5). Mortality risk was reduced by 19% in the treatment group.

However it should be mentioned that the control group feeding was higher in long-chain fat than most standard feedings (i.e. septic patients with ARDS (acute respiratory distress syndrome) can be fed standard diets with either a low total fat content or a high-fat content that is largely medium-chain fatty acid, and it is unknown how these diets would compare with the n-3 fatty acid feeding) and the results could not be replicated in a larger study. The n-3 fatty acid in this study was delivered in bolus fashion twice daily rather than by continuous infusion as part of a feeding regimen, and this could be an important difference influencing the outcomes. Furthermore, the two feeding formulas were not as similar to one another in terms of carbohydrate, fat, and protein, leaving open the possibility that other dietary differences in the studies interfered with the results.

Several evidence-based nutrition support guidelines for critically ill patients have concluded that enteral feeding formulas with n-3 fatty acids should be used in patients with acute respiratory distress syndrome. Some of these guidelines extend that recommendation to sepsis and more general critical care populations.

Metabolic dysregulation in critically ill patients

The changes in metabolism and nutrient requirement brought about by the inflammatory response to critical illness are thought to be adaptive, liberating fuels and stimulating pathways to produce glucose, acute phase proteins, and other components to return the patient to homeostasis. However, if infection intervenes, or other insults are sustained, the carefully orchestrated interplay between pro-inflammatory and anti-inflammatory signals that comprise the inflammatory response can become dysregulated and actually cause tissue damage leading to shock and organ failure. In such patients metabolism also becomes dysregulated, characterized by a further increase in catabolic rate, hyperglycemia, hypertrigly-ceridemia, and sometimes increased energy expenditure (although the change in energy expenditure still seems to follow changes in body temperature and minute ventilation). Provision of carbohydrate and fat are made more problematic by these changes. A higher portion of dietary protein is used ineffectively in some of these patients so that improvements in nitrogen balance are not realized from increasing the protein intake. If this metabolic defect occurs there seems to be a detrimental effect on outcome. The organ damage resulting from hyperinflamma-tory states may limit the tolerance to feeding, although with proper organ support the impact can be minimized. Nutrient intake in these patients should be charac-terized by increased protein intake, using urinary nitrogen loss when possible to determine if nitrogen balance is improved. Carbohydrate intake should be coordinated with insulin dosing to ensure that blood glucose does not exceed

150 mg/dL. A change in fat intake to an n-3 fatty acid based mixture should be considered, and minimizing negative energy deficits seems to be important.

Feeding routes and energy and protein requirements

One important area of disagreement in the recommendations of the published guidelines is the role of supplemental parenteral nutrition for patients who cannot be fed enterally or whose enteral feeding cannot be advanced to goal because of gastrointestinal intolerance. The ASPEN (American Society of Parenteral and Enteral Nutrition) guideline reserves early use of parenteral nutrition to patients with pre-existing malnutrition and inability to use enteral nutrition. If nutritional status is adequate, parenteral nutrition should not be considered until after 5 to 7 days inability to feed enterally. The Canadian guideline refrains from making a recommendation on the use of supplemental parenteral nutrition but does emphasize several strategies to maximize enteral feeding so that supplemental parenteral nutrition does not need to be considered. The European guideline on the other hand supports the early use of parenteral nutrition as a supplement to tube feeding if the tube feeding cannot be advanced. A recent study published after all of the guidelines seems to support the early use of parenteral nutrition to supplement enteral feeding if enteral feeding cannot be advanced. A randomized clinical trial was conducted on 275 patients started on early enteral feeding. On day 3 the patients were randomized to continue enteral feeding alone or to be supplemented with parenteral nutrition. Energy demand was determined by indirect calorimetry. Energy intake from day 4 to day 8 was 73 ± 27 vs $100 \pm 16\%$ of target in the enteral vs supplemental parenteral nutrition group. Being in the supplemental parenteral nutrition group reduced the risk of new infection, reduced antibiotic use, reduced the hours of mechanical ventilation, and reduced length of stay in the critical care unit. This study not only is evidence for the use of supplemental parenteral nutrition in the first week of critical care but is also further evidence favoring achievement of energy and protein intake targets.

Summary points

- Nutrition plays an important role in improving outcomes in critically ill patients.
- Evidence is accumulating that reaching protein and energy balance carries important benefits to these patients, including less infection, shorter length of stay, and reduced mortality.
- Energy requirements are predictable in about 75% of patients. It is not known whether this is sufficient accuracy or whether indirect calorimetry should be the standard way of determining energy needs. If indirect calorimetry is to be used, it needs to be repeated every 3 to 4 days to be more accurate than estimation methods.

- Precise protein requirements are not well established, with recommendations ranging from 1.5 to 2.5 g/kg body weight, and also recommending different body weights to use for the calculations in obese patients (ideal body weight vs. metabolically active body weight).
- Monitoring nitrogen balance may be the ideal way to determine whether protein intake is adequate in individual patients.
- In the critically ill patient water intake depends on the pathogenesis and severity of the acute insult and fluid needs can change as the illness evolves.

Further reading

Bartlett RH, Dechert RE, Mault JR, et al. Measurement of metabolism in multiple organ failure. Surgery 1982;92:771–779.

Burge JC, Goon A, Choban PS, Flancbaum L. Efficacy of hypocaloric total parenteral nutrition in hospitalized obese patients: a prospective, double-blind randomized trial. J Parenter Enteral Nutr 1994;18:203–207.

Frankenfield DC. Energy expenditure and protein requirements after traumatic injury. Nutr Clin Pract 2006;21:430–437.

Frankenfield DC. Validation of a metabolic rate equation in older obese critically ill people. J Parenter Enteral Nutr 2011;35:264–269.

Frankenfield DC, Smith JS, Cooney RN, Blosser SA. Relative association of fever and injury with hypermetabolism in critically ill patients. Injury 1997;28:617–621.

Frankenfield DC, Smith JS, Cooney RN. Accelerated nitrogen loss after traumatic injury is not attenuated by achievement of energy balance. J Parenter Enteral Nutr 1997;21:324–329.

Frankenfield DC. Energy expenditure and protein requirements after traumatic injury. Nutr Clin Pract 2006;21:430–437.

Frankenfield DC, Schubert A, Alam S, Cooney RN. Validation study of predictive equations for resting metabolic rate in critically ill patients. J Parenter Enteral Nutr 2009;33:27–36.

Frankenfield DC, Ashcraft CM, Galvan DA. Longitudinal assessment of metabolic rate in critically ill patients. J Parenter Enteral Nutr 2012;36:700–712.

Heidegger CP, Graf S, Thibault R, et al. Supplemental parenteral nutrition (SPN) in intensive care unit (ICU) patients for optimal energy coverage: improved clinical outcome. Clin Nutr 2011;1(S):2–3.

McClave SA, Martindale RG, Vanek VW, et al. Guidelines for the provision and assessment of nutrition support therapy in the adult critically ill patient. Society for Critical Care Medicine, American Society for Parenteral and Enteral Nutrition. J Parenter Enteral Nutr 2009;33:277–316.

Muller MJ, Bosy-Westphal A, Kutzner D, Heller M. Metabolically active components of fat-free mass and resting energy expenditure in humans: recent lessons from imaging technologies. Obes Rev 2002;3:113–122.

Pontes-Arruda A, Aragao AM, Albuquerque JD. Effects of enteral feeding with eicosapentaenoic acid, gamma-linolenic acid, and antioxidants in mechanically ventilated patients with severe sepsis and septic shock. Crit Care Med 2006;34:2325–2333.

Rice TW, Wheeler AP, Thompson BT, et al. Enteral omega-3 fatty acid, gamma-linolenic acid, and antioxidant supplementation in acute lung injury. J Am Med Assoc 2011;306:1574–1581.

Scheinkestel CD, Kar L, Marshall K, et al. Prospective randomized trial to assess caloric and protein needs of critically ill, anuric, ventilated patients requiring continuous renal replacement therapy. Nutrition 2003;19:909–916.

Shaw JHF, Wildbore M, Wolfe RR. Whole-body protein kinetics in severely septic patients: the response to glucose infusion and total parenteral nutrition. Ann Surg 1987;205:288–294.

Singer P, Anbar R, Cohen J, et al. The tight calorie control study (TICACOS): a prospective randomized clinical pilot study of nutrition support in critically ill patients. Intensive Care Med 2011;37:601–609.

Weijs PJM, Stapel SN, de Groot SDW, et al. Optimal protein and energy nutrition decreases mortality in mechanically ventilated, critically ill patients: a prospective observational cohort study. J Parenter Enteral Nutr 2012;36:60–68.

Wolfe RR, Goodenough RD, Burke JF, et al. Response of protein and urea kinetics in burn patients to different levels of protein intake. Ann Surg 1983;197:163–171.

Nutritional assessment of the critically ill patient

Mario Siervo and Carla Prado

Introduction

Nutrition plays a vital role in critical care since it can not only preserve or restore energy reserves but can also counter metabolic derangements commonly observed in critically ill patients. Protein energy malnutrition (PEM) in these patients is associated with increased morbidity with greater lengths of hospital stay and increased health costs ultimately also affecting survival. Proper nutrition directly reflects cell, organ, and system function as well as tissue healing, which has therefore a direct effect on the ability of patients to overcome the acute stressor and re-establish a normal health status.

Nutritional assessment aims to identify patients at higher risk of mortality and morbidity by discerning the ethiopathogenetic causes, which can guide the adoption of more effective nutritional strategies. Defined nutritional assessment protocols are also necessary to assess the effects of therapeutic plans on recovery rates and long-term prognosis. This risk-stratified approach may improve prognosis and it is associated with a more effective allocation of staff and financial resources.

Assessment of nutritional status

Acute critical illnesses complicate the interpretation of nutritional indexes and biomarkers because of the confounding effects of the disease process and aggressive treatments. An early nutritional assessment is required to achieve an accurate diagnosis of the level of malnutrition and identify patients in urgent need of nutritional therapy, thereby permitting adequate intervention to maximize recovery and/or maintenance of the patient's health status. Particularly important is the assessment of fluid and food intake. The identification of patients who will be able to resume oral feeding compared to patients needed to be assigned to more

Nutrition in Critical Care, ed. Peter Faber and Mario Siervo. Published by Cambridge University Press. © Cambridge University Press 2014.

aggressive treatments (enteral, parenteral) is a critical step in the risk stratification algorithm in critically ill patients. We would also like to emphasize the adoption of a multi-disciplinary, systematic approach to nutritional risk assessment to provide more accurate prognostic information.

Physical examination

The physical exam is important to assess the nutritional status as it offers the possibility of a direct interaction with the patient including evaluation of physical signs and symptoms as well as the individual psychological reaction to the disease and therapy. This is particularly important during treatment to monitor the recovery of the patients. The physical examination to assess nutritional status should consider the following signs and symptoms:
- Body size and shape (underweight, obesity, spine curvature)
- Mobility (strength, coordination)
- Autonomic functions (eating and swallowing, micturition, bowel movements)
- Skin (discoloration, contusions, lesions and edema, presence of pressure sores)
- Body temperature and breathing patterns
- Oral health
- Nausea, vomiting, diarrhea

The severity and type of modifications of these physical signs and symptoms vary between disorders and more detailed information is provided in other chapters in this book.

Anthropometry

Body weight is the sum of all body components (total body water, fat mass, muscular mass, bone mineral mass) and its measurement may be used as a proxy of individual's energy stores whereas changes in body weight may reflect shifts in energy balance. Body mass index (BMI) may represent a better indicator of nutritional status as it adjusts for body size of the individual but it is still not able to provide information on the single body composition components. Normal weight is defined as a BMI between 18.5 and 24.9 kg/m^2, whereas a BMI lower than 16 kg/m^2 is indicative of severe malnutrition and associated with a significant increase in mortality. Obesity is defined as a BMI greater than 30 kg/m^2 but morbid obesity (BMI > 40 kg/m^2) is certainly becoming more prevalent in the general population, which imposes additional logistic and medical challenges on the implementation of immediate and post-recovery nutritional therapies. A very important prognostic factor is unintentional weight loss but it may be difficult to determine the real loss of body mass in very sick individuals due to the poor accuracy of its measurement. This information may be obtained from a family member. Fluid therapy or edema may also mask weight changes and, again, relatives may be questioned in regard to change in body size or weight history. Waist circumference appears to have minimal additional prognostic value whereas other anthropometric variables, such as arm muscle circumference, may represent a useful indicator of malnutrition, which also has the additional advantage of low between-operator variability.

Nutritional questionnaires

These standardized tools are mostly used for a rapid diagnostic screening of patients at risk of complications and are therefore useful to initiate targeted nutritional treatments. The Subjective Global Assessment (SGA) is the most commonly used questionnaire for its simplicity, low cost, and high sensitivity and specificity. The administration of the SGA can be carried out in a few minutes and it is based on the assessment of clinical and dietary history as well as information obtained from the physical examination. The main components assessed by the SGA are: (1) food intake and underlying factors that may affect dietary intake and behavior; (2) weight history; (3) presence of gastrointestinal symptoms including frequency, intensity, and duration of the abnormalities. The nutrition-orientated physical examination also allows an indirect evaluation of energy balance, derived from the assessment of subcutaneous fat, muscle tone, and presence of excess fluids. The SGA is not only a diagnostic tool, but also identifies risk of complications and information on the most suitable feeding protocol. The accuracy of the SGA may be dependent on the clinical experience of the observer and on the lack of quantitative criteria used for monitoring the clinical parameters. Various other nutritional tools have been validated as screening methods in critical care such as the Malnutrition Universal Screening Tool (MUST), Mini Nutritional Assessment (MNA), Malnutrition Screening Tool (MST), Nutritional Risks Screening 2002 (NRS-2002), Nutrition Risk Index (NRI), and the Short Nutritional Assessment Questionnaire (SNAQ). The choice of the most suitable questionnaire may depend on several factors including the clinical conditions of the patient, availability of resources, level of training of staff, and, most importantly, the sensitivity and specificity of the questionnaire.

Biochemical indicators

Laboratory biomarkers help to assess the nutritional status by providing objective measurements closely related to specific physiological functions such as inflammation, glycemic control, electrolyte imbalance, and organ and system failures. The high level of precision of these measurements offers the advantage of monitoring the effects of nutritional interventions. For example, a decrease of serum concentrations of proteins may be a good indicator of protein energy malnutrition. However, it is important to note that there are many factors that may modify the concentration of serum proteins (hydration status, liver and kidney disease, increased catabolism, infection or inflammation, therapeutic administration) so the method should not be used exclusively for nutritional diagnosis. The most commonly used biochemical indicators of nutritional status are described in Table 2.1.

Table 2.1 Biochemical indicators of nutritional status

Biomarker	Comment
Albumin	Most frequent biochemical parameter for nutritional assessment. Low serum albumin concentrations are associated with higher occurrence of complications, mortality, and morbidity. Limitations: poor accuracy if assessed alone
Pre-albumin	Synthesized in the liver and partially catabolized in the kidneys. Levels are decreased in energy-protein malnutrition. Levels are decreased in conditions such as infection and hepatic failure, as well as in response to cytokines and hormones, and increased in renal failure
Transferrin	Beta-globulin; hepatic synthesis and involved in iron transportation. Transferrin is characterized by low sensitivity and specificity and its levels are increased in iron deficiency anemia and decreased in liver diseases, sepsis, malabsorption and inflammation
Retinol carrier protein	Short half-life (12 hours); levels increase with intake of vitamin A, decrease in hepatic disease, infection, and severe stress
Insulin-like growth factor (IGF-1)	Low molecular weight peptide, mediator of the growth hormone action. Used to assess the intensity of metabolic response to nutritional feeding protocols. Cost and complexity for the determination may limit its use. It decreases during the acute stages of inflammatory diseases
Creatinine-height index	During malnutrition and hyper-catabolic states, the degradation of skeletal muscle may be assessed by the measurement of urinary creatinine. Interpretation may be complicated by interfering factors such as age, stress, dietary protein content, and renal function. It requires 24-hour urine collection
3-methylhistidine	Metabolite resulting from muscle protein catabolism. Levels increase in hyper-catabolic states and decrease in older and undernourished subjects
Nitrogen balance	A non-invasive and accessible technique obtained from the difference between intake and excreted nitrogen. It is a good parameter to assess protein intake and catabolism and therefore repletion of malnourished patients (follow-up and monitoring of treatment).

Other biochemical parameters

Low serum cholesterol levels (<160 mg/dL) may be observed in malnourished patients but the sensitivity of this index may be low as a decrease may only be evident in more severe cases. A decrease in total lymphocyte count and decrease or absence (anergy) of cell immune response to specific antigens have been used as parameters for the assessment of nutritional status. However, the sensitivity of these indicators may again be low as they are influenced by various diseases and drugs such as infections, uremia, acidosis, cirrhosis, hepatitis, trauma, and surgical procedures. High glucose levels seem to be associated with an increased risk of complications and mortality. Controversial results have been obtained in recent trials suggesting that the impact of glucose control on clinical outcome may depend on the diabetic status of the patient as well as the risk of hypoglycemia. Therefore, feeding regimes and pharmacological therapeutic protocols should aim to maintain glucose levels around 10 mmol/L and avoid hypoglycemic events.

Indirect calorimetry

This method is considered the gold standard for the measurement of resting energy requirements in the critically ill patient. The method is based on the measurement of flow and concentration of inspired and expired oxygen and carbon dioxide, which allows the calculation of energy expenditure as well as macronutrient oxidation (protein, fat, carbohydrates). The evaluation of energy requirements in critically ill patients is mostly based on the application of predictive equations (e.g., Harris–Benedict, Mifflin) which may be largely inaccurate and introduce significant errors in the design of a nutritional therapy regimen. These errors should also be interpreted in the context of the current obesity epidemic as the magnitude of the error is directly associated with BMI. Therefore, the measurement of energy requirements using indirect calorimetry should be promoted in ICU, as the error of predictive equations is high and may affect the identification of the appropriate goals of nutritional therapies.

Monitoring of nutritional status

There is a general consensus that the nutritional status of critically ill patients should be frequently monitored to evaluate the effects of therapeutic protocols and progression of the disease. However, a full understanding of the evolution of the nutritional changes occurring during the acute and recovery phases of critically ill patients is far from being achieved. As previously suggested the screening methods should be chosen according to specific factors (type of disease, age, treatments) to enhance predictive power, accuracy, and limit inter-observer viability. This may be frequently repeated to detect the incidence of new malnutrition cases, particularly during prolonged hospital stays of 2 weeks or more. After the initiation of nutritional protocols, plasmatic electrolytes, glucose and magnesium, urea, creatinine, calcium, and inorganic phosphorus may be required to be checked daily until stabilization whereas total proteins, albumin, and pre-albumin may be less frequent (weekly). After the critical stage continued monitoring of these biochemical parameters should be performed. The reassessment of resting energy expenditure by indirect calorimetry can also be useful to adjust energy intake during the recovery phase to avoid overfeeding.

Conclusions

The assessment of nutritional status in critically ill patients is dynamic and rapidly changing in relation to the progression of the disease as well as to aggressive nutritional and pharmacological treatments. Therefore, the accuracy of single nutritional indicators for risk stratification and monitoring of critically ill patients is limited and data from several sources (medical history, physical examination, body composition, laboratory biomarkers) should be considered for an accurate assessment of nutritional status.

Summary points

- Nutritional assessment is a fundamental step in the management of critically ill patients.
- Acute critical illnesses complicate the interpretation of nutritional indexes and biomarkers because of the confounding effects of the disease process and aggressive treatments.
- An early nutritional assessment is required to achieve different diagnoses of malnutrition levels and identify patients in need of nutritional therapy, thereby permitting adequate intervention to support the recovery of ill patients.
- The adoption of a multi-disciplinary, systematic approach to nutritional risk assessment is essential to provide more accurate prognostic information.
- There is a general consensus that the nutritional status of critically ill patients should be frequently performed to evaluate the effects of therapeutic protocols and progression of the disease.

Further reading

Fontes D, Generoso SD, Toulson Davisson Correia MI. Subjective global assessment: a reliable nutritional assessment tool to predict outcomes in critically ill patients. Clin Nutr 2013 May 13. doi:pii: S0261–5614(13)00143-X.

Heyland DK, Dhaliwal R, Jiang X, Day AG. Identifying critically ill patients who benefit the most from nutrition therapy: the development and initial validation of a novel risk assessment tool. Crit Care 2011;15(6):R268.

Hiesmayr M. Nutrition risk assessment in the ICU. Curr Opin Clin Nutr Metab Care 2012;15(2):174–180.

Higgins PA, Daly BJ, Lipson AR, Su-Er G. Assessing nutritional status in chronically ill adult patients. Am J Crit Care 2006;15:1–99.

Kondrup J, Allison SP, Elia M, Vellas B, Plauth M. Educational and Clinical Practice Committee, European Society of Parenteral and Enteral Nutrition (ESPEN). ESPEN guidelines for nutritional screening 2002. Clin Nutr 2003;22(4):415–421.

McClave SA, Martindale RG, Kiraly L. The use of indirect calorimetry in the intensive care unit. Curr Opin Clin Nutr Metab Care 2013;16(2):202–208.

Prins A. Nutritional assessment of the critically ill patient. S Afr J Clin Nutr 2010;23 (1):11–18.

Rodriguez L. Nutritional status: assessing and understanding its value in the critical care setting. Crit Care Nurs Clin North Am 2004;16(4):509–514.

Sungurtekin H, Sungurtekin U, Okke D. Nutrition assessment in critically ill patients. Nutr Clin Pract 2008;23(6):635–641.

Thibault R, Pichard C. Nutrition and clinical outcome in intensive care patients. Curr Opin Clin Nutr Metab Care 2010;13(2):177–183.

3

Body composition assessment of the critically ill patient

Ying Ji and Dympna Gallagher

Introduction

Patients who are critically ill frequently experience weight loss that consists of losses in fat and lean mass stores. In some instances, depending on the underlying illness (e.g., advanced cachexia, liver cirrhosis, renal failure, and heart failure), weight loss may not in fact be evident as it is masked by fluid retention. The latter can result in a delay in providing the patient with the appropriate nutritional intervention. In the presence of malnutrition, sarcopenia, cachexia, heightened inflammatory response, hypermetabolic state, or any combination of these, there is an accelerated loss in lean tissue stores including skeletal muscle mass. Knowledge therefore of body composition is critical to providing the appropriate nutritional intervention.

Body composition measurement methods vary in complexity and precision, and range from simple field-based methods (anthropometry, bioimpedance analysis) to more technically challenging laboratory-based methods (dual-energy x-ray absorptiometry, hydrostatic weighing, air plethysmography, whole-body counting for ^{40}K, deuterium and bromide dilutions, and magnetic resonance imaging).

Factors that influence body composition

Fat mass

Infants average about 10–15% fat at birth. This increases to about 30% by 6 months of age and then begins to gradually decline during early childhood. Total body fat continues to increase during adolescence. Percent body fat increases in girls between 9 and 20 years but decreases in boys after 13 years as fat-free mass (FFM) rapidly increases. Total body fat mass increases slowly with age during

Nutrition in Critical Care, ed. Peter Faber and Mario Siervo. Published by Cambridge University Press. © Cambridge University Press 2014.

adulthood. Assuming that the body consists of two compartments, fat and fat-free mass (body weight =fat + fat-free mass), the reference percent fat for adults is age, race, and sex dependent.

Sex differences in body composition are present at birth with females having greater body fat than males. These differences become more pronounced during the adolescent spurt and sexual maturation. Differences reflect a larger fat-free mass, total bone mineral content (especially of the limb skeleton), and skeletal muscle mass in males and greater percent body fat in females. The sex differences established during adolescence persist through adulthood and there is a sex difference in changes in specific components of body composition with advancing age.

Fat-free mass increases during growth, is relatively stable throughout maturity, and declines during senescence. Total body bone mass is a component of fat-free mass that increases with age during growth and development to maturity, reaching peak bone mass between 20 and 30 years of age and then decreases with age after reaching a peak. There is an accelerated loss of bone mineral density in women and men greater than 50 years of age that is hormonally related. Skeletal muscle mass is another component of fat-free mass. In general, growth and development are stages of rapid accretion of skeletal muscle with marked sexual dimorphism developing during adolescence. Skeletal muscle mass is relatively stable within individuals during adulthood up to about age 30 to 40 years, after which mass begins to decrease. A third component of fat-free mass is the body organs. The brain and liver are the largest organs in the body, making up about 12.2% and 4.5% of total body weight at birth respectively. These percentages decrease during maturity until around 20 years of age and remain stable over most of the life span. Kidneys and heart are the next largest organs, comprising respectively about 0.45% and 0.54% of body weight during adulthood. The available data suggest slight decreases with age in the relative sizes of these organs beginning in middle age and progressing into senescence.

Skeletal muscle mass

Skeletal muscle mass (SM) represents ~40% of body weight in healthy young adults. SM mass decreases to ~30% of young adult values at elderly ages. SM mass represents ~60% of the body's cell mass. Two components are usually considered as representative of whole-body metabolically active tissue, body cell mass and fat-free mass (FFM = body weight – fat mass). SM is one of the more difficult components to quantify. Common measurement methods include anthropometry, dual-energy x-ray absorptiometry (DXA) derived appendicular skeletal muscle (ASM), and magnetic resonance imaging (MRI). In disease and critically ill states, a measure of skeletal muscle mass is frequently desired for nutritional intervention purposes.

Choice of body composition methods

Body mass index

The body mass index (BMI = weight kg/height m^2) continues to be the most commonly used index of weight status, where normal weight is a BMI 18.5–25.9 kg/m^2, overweight is a BMI 25.0–29.9 kg/m^2, and obese a BMI ≥ 30.0 kg/m^2. Despite BMI not being a measure of body composition, it is commonly considered an index of fatness due to the high correlation between BMI and percent body fat in children and adults. The prediction of percent body fat in African-American (AA), Asian (As), and Caucasian (C) adults was found to vary by age (higher in older persons), sex (higher in males), and race (higher in As compared to AA and C). The following equation is proposed to estimate percent body fat:

$$\text{Percent Body Fat} = 76.0 - 1097 \times (1/\text{BMI}) - 20.6 \times \text{SEX} + 0.053 \\ \times \text{Age} + 95.0 \times \text{Asian} \times (1/\text{BMI}) - 0.044 \\ \times \text{Asian} \times \text{Age} + 154 \times \text{SEX} \times (1/\text{BMI}) \\ + 0.034 \times \text{SEX} \times \text{Age},$$

where sex = 0 for female and 1 for male; race = 1 for Asian, 2 for other races.

In an analysis including Hispanic-American (HA) adults, no differences in the prediction of percent fat from BMI were observed between HA, European-American (EA), and AA men. In women, differences in percent body fat predicted by BMI were observed between HA and EA ($P < 0.002$) and AA and HA ($P = 0.020$), but not between AA and EA ($P = 0.490$). At BMIs < 30 kg/m^2, HA tended to have more body fat than EA and AA, and at BMIs > 35 kg/m^2, EA tended to have more body fat than the other groups.

Anthropometry

For routine clinical use, anthropometric measurements have been preferred due to ease of measurement and low cost. Waist circumference and the waist-hip ratio measurements are commonly used surrogates of fat distribution, especially in epidemiology studies. Waist circumference is highly correlated with visceral fat and is included as a clinical risk factor in the definition of the metabolic syndrome. Specifically, waist circumferences greater than 102 cm (40 in) in men and greater than 88 cm (35 in) in women are suggestive of elevated risk.

Prediction of percent fat and/or fat-free mass

Skinfold thicknesses which estimate the thickness of the subcutaneous fat layer are highly correlated with percent body fat. Since the subcutaneous fat layer varies in thickness throughout the body, a combination of site measures is recommended, reflecting upper and lower body distribution. Predictive percent body fat equations based on skinfold measures are age and sex specific in adults and children. Examples of predictive equations include Jackson–Pollock and Durnin–Womersley in adults, and Boileau and Bray et al. in children.

Prediction of skeletal muscle mass

Arm, thigh, and calf muscle areas can be estimated based on skinfold thickness and limb circumference measures. In one study, a skinfold-circumference model was found to have a higher accuracy than a body weight and height model in predicting total body SM in healthy adult populations. The following two equations are proposed to estimate skeletal muscle and these models were developed and cross-validated in non-obese healthy adults (BMI < 30 kg/m^2). These measurements can be applied in both ambulatory and non-ambulatory patients.

Model 1

$$\text{SM} = \text{Ht} \times (0.00744 \times \text{CAG}(2) + 0.00088 \times \text{CTG}(2) + 0.00441$$
$$\times \text{CCG}(2)) + 2.4 \times \text{sex} - 0.048 \times \text{age} + \text{race} + 7.8$$

where $R^2 = 0.91$; $P < 0.0001$; SEE = 2.2 kg; sex = 0 for female and 1 for male; race = −2.0 for Asian, 1.1 for African-American, and 0 for Caucasian and Hispanic; Ht is height in meters; CAG = skinfold corrected upper arm girth; CTG = skinfold corrected thigh girth; CCG = skinfold corrected calf girth; all girth measurements in centimeters.

Model 2

$$\text{SM} = 0.244 \times \text{BW} + 7.80 \times \text{Ht} + 6.6 \times \text{sex} - 0.098 \times \text{age}$$
$$+ \text{race} - 3.3$$

where $R^2 = 0.86$, $P: < 0.0001$, and SEE = 2.8 kg; sex = 0 for female and 1 for male, race = −1.2 for Asian, 1.4 for African-American, and 0 for Caucasian and Hispanic; BW is body weight in kilograms, and Ht is height in meters.

Bioimpedance analysis (BIA)

BIA is a simple, low-expense, non-invasive body composition measurement method. BIA is based on the electrical conductive properties of the human body. Measures of bioelectrical conductivity are proportional to total body water and the body's components with high water concentrations such as fat-free and skeletal muscle mass. BIA assumes that the body consists of two compartments, fat and fat-free mass (body weight = fat + fat-free mass). BIA is best known as a technique for the measurement of percent body fat. Compared to multi-compartment body composition models, a two-compartment model approach

(BIA and anthropometry being two examples) produces greater errors when estimating percent body fat in children and adults. Several selected single-frequency BIA equations for predicting fat-free mass have been published in different age groups. No single equation has been validated in all groups.

It is reported that there is a strong correlation between BIA resistance and skeletal muscle measurements in the arms and legs. Janssen et al. reported that MRI-measured SM mass is strongly correlated to the BIA resistance index (Ht^2/R) and the following SM prediction equation was developed from a multi-ethnic group (Caucasian, Hispanic, and African-American) of females (n = 158) and males (n = 230):

$$SM\ mass\ (kg) = \left[(Ht^2/R \times 0.401) + (sex \times 3.825) + (age \times -0.071)\right] + 5.102$$

where Ht is height in centimeters; R is BIA resistance in ohms; sex = 0 for female and 1 for male; age in years; R^2 = 0.86; SEE = 2.7 kg (9%).

Dual-energy x-ray absorptiometry (DXA)

DXA provides an important means of quantifying total body and regional fat mass, skeletal muscle mass, and bone mineral mass and density. Using specific anatomic landmarks, the trunk, legs, and arms are identified. The fat-free soft tissue (i.e., nonfat, nonbone mineral mass) of the extremities is largely (~76%) skeletal muscle and is considered ASM mass. DXA- and MRI-measured lower limb SM mass have been shown to be highly correlated (r = 0.94, P < 0.001) in adults and high correlations have been found between DXA-measured ASM and MRI-derived total body skeletal muscle mass in adults (r = 0.98).

Baumgartner et al. developed an anthropometric equation for predicting ASM mass in elderly Hispanic and non-Hispanic white men and women. Sarcopenia was defined as ASM (kg)/height^2 (m^2) less than two standard deviations below the mean of the young reference group. In the elderly men, the mean ASM/height^2 was approximately 87% of the young group. The corresponding value in women was approximately 80%. Obese and sarcopenic persons are reported as having worse outcomes than those who are non-obese and sarcopenic.

Magnetic resonance imaging

There is strong support for the use of MRI as a reference method for evaluating and monitoring changes over time in whole-body and regional body composition. Due to the expense associated with this technique, it does not present as a practical measurement method for use in clinical screening. However, it needs to be acknowledged that in vivo measurement in humans of SM mass, total adipose tissue (TAT) mass and its distribution, and masses of several organs is possible. SM and TAT, including total subcutaneous adipose tissue (SAT), visceral adipose tissue (VAT), and intermuscular adipose tissue (IMAT), can be measured using whole-body multi-slice MRI. Subjects are placed on the scanner platform with their arms extended above their heads. The protocol involves the acquisition of approximately 40 axial images, 10 mm thickness, and at 40 mm intervals across the whole body. Image analysis software is used to analyze images on a PC. MRI-volume estimates are converted to mass using the assumed density of 1.04 kg/L for SM and 0.92 kg/L for adipose tissue. The technical error values for repeated measurements of the same scan by the same observer of MRI-derived SM, SAT, VAT, and IMAT volumes in our laboratory are 1.9%, 0.96%, 1.97%, and 0.65%, respectively.

Measuring changes in body composition

During the adult life span, body weight generally increases slowly and progressively until about the seventh decade, when it declines into old age. An increased incidence of physical disabilities and co-morbidities are likely linked to aging-associated body composition changes. Characterization of the aging processes has identified losses in muscle mass, force, and strength, which collectively are defined as 'sarcopenia'. Little is known about the overall rate at which sarcopenia develops in otherwise healthy elderly subjects, whether this rate of progression differs between women and men, and the underlying mechanisms responsible for age-related sarcopenia.

We have shown that there is an accelerated rate of skeletal muscle mass loss in the presence of weight stability over a 2-year period in healthy independently living, ambulatory elderly African-American females (mean age at baseline 75.5 ± 5.1). Body composition was measured using repeated multi-slice MRI and DXA. Despite no significant changes in body weight ($P = 0.62$) or FFM ($P = 0.6$), SM mass ($P = 0.02$) and bone mineral content decreased ($P = 0.03$) and IMAT ($P < 0.001$) and VAT increased ($P = 0.01$) after adjusting for their baseline values. No changes were found in physical performance (200 m walk; 2 minute walk), function (chair rise), or activity (physical activity scale for the elderly), grip strength, or standing balance. These data demonstrate a disproportionate loss of SM over a 2-year period in healthy elderly subjects.

Acknowledgment

This work was supported by grants RO1-DK72507, UO1-DK094463, and P30-DK26687 from the National Institutes of Health.

Summary points

- It is important to recognize that there is no single measurement method in existence that is error free. Furthermore, bias can be introduced if a

Table 3.1 Available measurement methods of body composition and energy expenditure in ambulatory and non-ambulatory patients

Method/main result(s)	Advantages	Disadvantages	Prediction equation
Anthropometry/body weight, height, skinfolds, body circumferences, and dimensions	Inexpensive, simple to acquire, safe, and can be used in settings that range from the research laboratories to field settings	The need for trained observers, relatively high between-measurement technical error for some measurements, mechanical limitations of some instruments for the very obese, "errors" in some geometric prediction models assuming stable between-subject anatomic proportions, and population specificity of component prediction formulas	(see below)

Predicting skeletal muscle mass[1]:

Skeletal muscle (kg) = BH (cm) × (0.00744 × CAG2 + 0.00088X CTG2 + 0.00088X CTG2 + 9.9941X CCG2 + 2.4X sex + race + 7.8)

CAG=corrected arm girth; CTG=corrected thigh girth; CCG=corrected calf girth;

Sex: 0 for female; 1 for male; race: 0=white/Hispanic, 1.1 for African-American, −0.2 for Asian

Skeletal muscle (kg) = 0.244 × BW + 7.80 × BH + 6.6 × sex −0.098 × age + race − 3.3

Sex=0 for female; 1 for male; race=−1.2 for Asian, 1.4 for African-American, and 0 for white and Hispanic

Predicting percent fat (%BF)/body density (BD)[2]:

Study	Race	Gender	Age (yrs)	Equation
Peterson et al. (2003)	Not Specified	Males	Adult	%BF = 20.94878 + (age × 0.1166) − (Ht × 0.11666) + (sum of 4 skinfolds × 0.42696) − ([sum of 4 skinfolds]2 × 0.00159) Sum of triceps + subscapular + suprailiac + midthigh
		Females	Adult	%BF = 22.18945 + (age × 0.06368) + (BMI × 0.60404) − (Ht × 0.14520) + (sum of 4 skinfolds × 0.30919) − ([sum of 4 skinfolds]2 × 0.00099562) Sum of triceps + subscapular + suprailiac + midthigh
Durnin & Wormersley (1974)	Not Specified	Males n = 209	17–72	BD = 1.1765 − 0.0744(log10X) X (mm) = Σ4 skinfolds (triceps, biceps, subscapular, iliac crest)
		Females n = 272	16–68	BD = 1.1567 − 0.0717(log10X) X (mm) = Σ4 skinfolds (triceps, biceps, subscapular, iliac crest)
Forsyth & Sinning (1973)	Not Specified	Males n = 50	19–22	BD = 1.10647 − 0.00162(X₁) − 0.00144(X₂) − 0.00077(X₃) + 0.00071(X₄) X₁ = subscapular skinfold (mm) X₂ = abdominal skinfold (mm) X₃ = triceps skinfold (mm) X₄ = mid-axilla skinfold (mm)
Jackson et al. (1980)	Not Specified	Females n = 249	18–55	BD = 1.24374 − 0.03162(log10X₁) − 0.0066(X₄) BD = 1.24389 − 0.04057(log10X₂) − 0.00016(X₃) X₁ = Σ₄ skinfolds (triceps, abdominal, front thigh, iliac crest in mm) X₂ = Σ₃ skinfolds (triceps, front thigh, iliac crest in mm)

Table 3.1 (cont.)

Method/main result(s)	Advantages	Disadvantages	Prediction equation			
			X_3 = age (yrs) X_4 = gluteal circumference (cm) $BD = 1.09665 - 0.00103(X_1) - 0.00056(X_2) - 0.00054(X_3)$			
			X_1 = triceps skinfold (mm) X_2 = subscapular skinfold (mm) X_3 = abdominal skinfold (mm)	Katch & McArdle (1973)	Caucasian	Males $n = 53$ 19.3 ± 1.5
			$BD = 1.09246 - 0.00049(X_1) - 0.00075(X_2) - 0.00710(X_3) - 0.00121(X_4)$			Females $n = 69$ 20.3 ± 1.8
			X_1 = subscapular skinfold (mm) X_2 = iliac crest skinfold (mm) X_3 = biepicondylar humerus breadth (cm) X_4 = thigh girth (cm)			
			$BD = 1.08543 - 0.000886(X_1) - 0.00040(X_2)$ X_1 = abdominal skinfold (mm) X_2 = front thigh skinfold (mm)	Wilmore & Behnke (1969)	Not Specified	Males $n = 133$ 22.04 ± 3.10
			$BD = 1.06234 - 0.00068(X_1) - 0.00039(X_2) - 0.00025(X_3)$ X_1 = subscapular skinfold (mm) X_2 = triceps skinfold (mm) X_3 = front thigh skinfold (mm)			Females $n = 128$ 21.41 ± 3.76

Selected single-frequency BIA equations for predicting fat-free mass[2]

Method/main result(s)	Advantages	Disadvantages	Prediction equation	Population			
Bioelectrical impedance analysis/resistance, stature	Inexpensive, portable, simple, safe, quick	All variables should be considered: hydration status, consumption of food or beverages, ambient air and skin temperatures, recent physical activity and bladder activity	Baumgartner et al. (1991)	White /USA	35M, 63F	65–94	$0.28(S2/R) + 0.27(W) + 4.5(S) + 0.31(\text{Thigh C}) - 1.732$
			Deurenberg et al. (1991)	Unknown /Netherland	661	16–83	$0.34(S2/R) - 0.127(\text{age}) + 0.273(W) + 4.56(\text{Sex}) + 15.34(S) - 12.44$
			Segal et al. (1985)	Unknown / USA	1069M	17–59	$0013(S2) - 0.044(R) + 0.305(W) - 0.168(\text{age}) + 22.668$
			Segal et al. (1988)	Unknown /USA	498F	17–62	$0.0011(S2) - 0.021(R) + 0.232(W) - 0.068(\text{age}) + 14.595$

Two and Three-Compartment Body Composition Models for measuring percentage fat (%Fat)[3]

Method/main result(s)	Advantages	Disadvantages	Model	Population	Equations for %Fat	Reference
Air displacement plethysmography/total body volume	Relatively high accuracy, fast	Many individuals with BMI > 60 kg/m² will not fit within the instrument	2C	General population	$100 \times (4.95/D_b - 4.50)$	Siri (1956)
			2C	Lean and obese	$100 \times (4.570/D_b - 4.142)$	Brozek et al. (1963)
			2C	African-American males	$100 \times (4.374/D_b - 3.928)$	Schutte (1984)
			2C	African-American females	$100 \times (4.83/D_b - 4.37)$	Ortiz et al. (1992)

D_b = Weight/Total Body Volume, body density (in kg/L)

Method	Advantages	Limitations	Four-Compartment Body Composition Models for measuring percentage fat (%Fat)[3]		
			Model	Equations for %Fat	Reference
DXA/total body bone mineral	Easy to use, low x-ray radiation exposure, accurate for limb lean and fat	Bias: body size, sex, fatness. Many individuals with BMI >40kg/m² will not fit within the field-of-view for soft tissue. Expensive equipment and specialized. Cannot be used in pregnant women	3C	$100 \times [6.386/D_b - 3.961 \times TBBM - 6.090]$	Lohman (1986)
			4C	$100 \times [2.747/D_b - 0.714 \times (TBW/W) + 1.129 \times TBBM/W - 2.037]$	Selinger (1977)
			4C	$100 \times [2.748/D_b - 0.6744 \times (TBW/W) + 1.4746 \times (TBBM/W) - 2.051]$	Heymsfield et al. (1990)
			4C	$100 \times [2.513/D_b - 0.739 \times (TBW/W) + 0.947 \times (TBBM/W) - 1.790]$	Withers et al. (1992)

D_b= Weight/Total Body Volume, body density (in kg/L); TBW, total body water (in kg); W, body weight (in kg); TBBM, total body bone mineral (osseous + non-osseous; in kg)

Dilution techniques /total body water by Oxygen-18 labeled water, extracellular water by bromide dilution	Acceptable in all age groups and body sizes. Easy to administer stable isotopes. Simple, relatively inexpensive, and easy to carry out even in isolated settings	Expensive equipment. Most approaches allow reliable measurement of TBW with a technical error in the range of 1% to 3%. Often require several hours and subject conditions can be very variable depending on hydration status, the presence of disease, or ambient conditions such as environmental temperature

Three-Compartment Body Composition Models for measuring percentage fat (%Fat)[3]

$\%Fat = 100 \times [2.118/Db \ 0.78 \times (TBW/W) \ 1.354]$ (Siri, 1961)

D_b= Weight/Total Body Volume, body density (in kg/L); TBW, total body water (in kg); W, body weight (in kg)

Whole-Body Counting	Systems are simple to operate. No recognized health risks	Costly installation. Extremely heavy equipment

SM prediction model[6]

$SM \ (kg) = 0.0085 \times TBK \ (mmol)$ (r_2 = 0.98, P<0.001)

$SM \ (kg) = 0.0093 \times TBK \ (mmol) - 1.31 \times sex + 0.59 \times black + 0.024 \times age - 3.21$ (sex is 0 for women and 1 for men, and black is 1 for African Americans and 0 for the other 3 ethnic groups; r_2 = 0.96, P<0.001; SEE = 1.52kg)

MRI	High accuracy and reproducibility for whole-body and regional adipose tissue and skeletal muscle	Many individuals with BMI >40kg/m² will not fit within the field-of-view for soft tissue. Expensive. Instrument access and the need for trained image analysis technicians may limit routine imaging method use to specialized research studies and centers

Regression equations to predict total visceral adipose tissue (VAT) volume from VAT area imaged at L4-L5 and at 6cm above L4-L5 (L4-L5 + 6)[7]

Variables in model	R^2
L4-L5*	0.8269
L4-L5*+sex*+race*	0.8678
L4-L5*+sex*+race*+age group†	0.8674
L4-L5*+sex*+race*+BMI*	0.8777
L4-L5*+sex*+race*+waist*	0.8843
L4-L5*+sex*+race*+age group*+ BMI† + waist*+(race × L4-L5)*+ (sex × L4-L5)*	0.8983
(L4-L5 + 6)*	0.9737
(L4-L5 + 6)*+sex*+race*	0.9741

Table 3.1 (cont.)

Variables in model	R^2
(L4-L5 + 6)*+sex*+race*+age group*	0.9745
(L4-L5 + 6)*+sex*+race*+age group*+BMI*	0.9750
(L4-L5 + 6)*+sex*+race*+age group*+BMI*+waist*	.9756
(L4-L5 + 6)*+sex*+ race† + age group*+ BMI†+ waist*+ (race × 6 cm)*+ (sex × 6cm)*	0.9766

R2, percentage of variance explained by the regression variables

* Term is significant in the model.

* Term is not significant in the model.

[1] Lee RC, Wang Z, Heo M, et al. (2000). Total-body skeletal muscle mass: development and cross-validation of anthropometric prediction models. Am J Clin Nutr 72(3):796–803.

[2] Heymsfield SB, Lohman TG, Wang Z, et al. (2005). Human Body Composition. Champaign, US: Human Kinetics.

[3] Roche AF, Heymsfield SB, Lohman TG. (1996). Human Body Composition, Human Kinetics.

[4] Schutte JE, Townsend EJ, Hugg J, et al. (1984). Density of lean body mass is greater in Blacks than in Whites. J Appl Physiol 56:1647–1649.

[5] Ortiz O, Russell M, Daley TL, et al. (1992). Differences in skeletal muscle and bone mineral mass between black and white females and their relevance to estimates of body composition. Am J Clin Nutr 55:8–13.

[6] Wang Z, Zhu S, Wang J, et al. (2003). Whole-body skeletal muscle mass: development and validation of total-body potassium prediction models. Am J Clin Nutr 77(1):76–82.

[7] Demerath EW, Shen W, Lee M, et al. (2007). Approximation of total visceral adipose tissue with a single magnetic resonance image. Am J Clin Nutr 85(2):362–368.

[8] Weissman C, Kemper M, Elwyn DH, et al. (1986). The energy expenditure of the mechanically ventilated critically ill patient: an analysis. Chest 89(2):254–259.

BH, body height; BW, body weight; BMI, body mass index; R, resistance; S, stature; W;;body weight; DXA, dual-energy x-ray absorptiometry; MRI, magnetic resonance imaging.

measurement method makes assumptions related to body composition proportions and characteristics that are inaccurate across different populations (for example, a method that was developed and validated in a healthy cohort and is then applied to a cohort with a disease).

- Some methodological concerns include the following: (1) hydration of fat-free body mass changes with disease progression or with medical/pharmacological intervention or treatment; (2) the density of fat-free body mass changes with age, disease progression, or with medical/pharmacological intervention or treatment; (3) skeletal muscle mass atrophy due to bed rest coupled with fluid retention both of which may be masked by little change in body weight
- These between-group differences influence the absolute accuracy of methods for estimating fatness or FFM involving the two-compartment model approach in diseased or critically ill states.

Further reading

Baracos VE, Reiman T, Mourtzakis M, et al. Body composition in patients with non-small cell lung cancer: a contemporary view of cancer cachexia with the use of computed tomography image analysis. Am J Clin Nutr 2010;91(4):1133S-1137S.

Binymin K, Herrick A, Carlson G, et al. The effect of disease activity on body composition and resting energy expenditure in patients with rheumatoid arthritis. J Inflamm Res 2011;4:61–66.

Brinksma A, Huizinga G, Sulkers E, et al. Malnutrition in childhood cancer patients: a review on its prevalence and possible causes. Crit Rev Oncol Hematol 2012;83(2):249–275.

Cao DX, Wu GH, Zhang B, et al. Resting energy expenditure and body composition in patients with newly detected cancer. Clin Nutr 2010;29(1):72–77.

Di Somma S, Gori CS, Grandi T, et al. Fluid assessment and management in the emergency department. Contrib Nephrol 2010;164:227–236.

Gallagher D, DeLegge M. Body composition (sarcopenia) in obese patients: implications for care in the intensive care unit. J Parenter Enteral Nutr 2011;35:21S

Heymsfield SB, Lohman TG, Wang Z, et al. *Human Body Composition*. Champaign, US: Human Kinetics; 2005.

Jiang F, Bo Y, Cui T, et al. Estimating the hydration status in nephrotic patients by leg electrical resistivity measuring method. Nephrology (Carlton) 2010;15(4):476–479.

Rozentryt P, von Haehling S, Lainscak M, et al. The effects of a high-caloric protein-rich oral nutritional supplement in patients with chronic heart failure and cachexia on quality of life, body composition, and inflammation markers: a randomized, double-blind pilot study. J Cachexia Sarcopenia Muscle 2010;1(1):35–42.

Thibault R, Cano N, Pichard C. Quantification of lean tissue losses during cancer and HIV infection/AIDS. Curr Opin Clin Nutr Metab Care 2011;14(3):261–267.

4

Micronutrient and vitamin physiology and requirements in critically ill patients

Timothy Eden, Minha Rajput-Ray, and Sumantra Ray

Introduction

Appropriate micronutrient therapy, both to meet physiological requirements as well as treat disease-related deficiencies, is of vital importance in critical care. It is important to recognize the individualized needs of the 'critically ill patient' and tailor both overall medical and nutritional management plans. Existing literature on this population group is limited by factors such as patient heterogeneity, sample sizes, and variability in baseline nutritional assessment. It is therefore important to ensure continuous evaluation of individual nutritional needs as there may be considerable departure from general recommendations.

A feature of the "critically ill patient" is the association with a catabolic stress state and the influence of the systemic inflammatory response. This is coupled with adjustments in requirements for macronutrients as well as micronutrients, secondary to altered physiological states such as infection and multi-organ dysfunction. The purpose of this chapter is to discuss and highlight relevant micronutrient and vitamin physiology and outline how these are altered in the critical care setting. The aim in this setting is to enable an adequate supply of micronutrients to ensure homeostatic, metabolic, and immune functions to optimize recovery with respect to the considerations below:

- Morbidity/mortality
- Infectious complications
- Length of ICU stay
- Overall hospital stay
- Acute phase response
- Oxidative stress
- Multi-organ dysfunction
- Preservation of lean body mass

Treatment goals

The key goals of nutrition therapy in critical care include the following:
- Modulation of the stress response and attenuating damage due to increased oxidative stress.

Nutrition in Critical Care, ed. Peter Faber and Mario Siervo. Published by Cambridge University Press. © Cambridge University Press 2014.

- Preservation of lean body mass/tissue.
- Ongoing assessment and monitoring to detect micronutrient deficiencies and initiate replacement when required.

At risk individuals

There are limited data on the inter-individual variation in micronutrient and vitamin requirements in the 'critically ill patient', or indeed specific supplementation recommendations to optimize recovery, decrease length of stay, and lower morbidity as well as mortality. However, it is well recognized that adequate provision of vitamins and trace elements plays a significant role in the delivery of any nutritional management plan in this setting. The role of the clinician thus needs to incorporate the identification of individuals at risk, determine the route of delivery, i.e., enteral nutrition (EN) or parenteral nutrition (PN), and prescribe feeds accordingly. Depletion of one or more micronutrient may have occurred prior to feeding or can result as the disease state progresses. Such deficiencies rarely occur in isolation and multiple factors determine the extent of progression/deficiency, as outlined below:

- Pre-admission nutritional status and the influence of malnutrition, disease-related anorexia, and times of inadequate ingestion or absorption of specific nutrients.
- Duration and severity of declining nutritional status while in the hospital setting secondary to surgery or other medical conditions and interventions impacting intake.
- Increased losses directly related to physiological state, e.g., small bowel fistula/aspirate (high in zinc), dialysis (increased losses of water-soluble vitamins), burn exudate (high in zinc, copper, and selenium), biliary fluid losses (high in copper).
- Underlying disease states influencing ingestion, digestion, and absorption – celiac disease, inflammatory bowel disease (IBD), alcoholism, or surgical intervention of the gastrointestinal (GI) tract impacting absorption.

Adult micronutrient requirements in critically ill patients

Providing micronutrients to include the full range of trace elements and vitamins in accordance with recommended daily allowances (RDAs) is an integral part of nutritional support in routine clinical practice. However, guidance specific to critical care utilizes the recommendations based on the Nutrition Advisory Group of the American Medical Association (AMA-NAG) which assumes elevated requirements in accordance with an altered physiological state.

Therefore in critical care, specific nutritional requirements have been recognized to increase secondary to multiple organ failure, increased oxidative stress, and patients becoming hyper-metabolic. More common acute deficiencies apparent in critical care and ICU care are listed below showing associated clinical manifestations:

- Thiamine (B_1) – leading to congestive cardiac failure, lactic acidosis.
- Vitamin C (ascorbic acid) – scurvy.
- Copper – arrhythmias, altered immunity, and pseudo-scurvy.
- Selenium – acute cardiomyopathy.
- Zinc – delayed wound healing and increased infection.

Other common observations within the ICU setting secondary to the acute phase response can include alterations to various plasma concentrations of micronutrients and are outlined below:

- ↓Iron as a result of ↑ferritin in the liver.
- ↓Zinc as a result of ↑metallothionein in liver.
- ↓Vitamin C (ascorbic acid) due to ↑transfer into tissues.
- ↑Copper due to ↑caeruloplasmin synthesis and release.
- ↓Selenium due to ↓selenoprotein P in plasma.
- ↓Vitamin A secondary to ↓retinol binding protein in plasma.

Monitoring of micronutrients

Due to the current lack of consensus guidance on the requirements of micronutrients in critical illness, this impacts on the rationale for clear monitoring guidelines in clinical practice. However, in cases where manifestations are indicative of deficiency, methods of assessment can be seen in Table 4.1 which summarizes corrective doses that may be needed to achieve optimal micronutrient and vitamin levels as well as taking into consideration the route of administration.

Absorption and interactions

Fat-soluble vitamins A, D, E, and K are poorly absorbed in individuals in whom fat absorption is depressed in certain disease states in turn leading to malabsorption, or less frequently, when overall fat intake is significantly decreased. Vitamins A, D, and E are primarily absorbed in the duodenum and the upper jejunum due to its links with fat digestion aided by bile and pancreatic lipase (Note: pancreatic insufficiencies and bile losses may therefore also impact absorption). Vitamin K absorption occurs further along the GI tract in the ascending colon. Water-soluble vitamins B1, B2, B3, B5, B6, biotin, and vitamin C are in most part absorbed in the jejunum via Na^+ co-transport. Folic acid and B12 are mainly absorbed in the ileum (Figure 4.1).

GI losses and chronic disease states are the most common etiological determinants of acute micronutrient deficiencies. In terms of GI losses high-output fistula and significant episodes of diarrhea can result in deficient states and should be monitored and corrected accordingly alongside the treatment of the root cause. Interactions between various vitamins can be additive but also have deleterious effects. Vitamins E and C are synergistic in nature whereby the latter helps to recycle the former and consequently in deficient states of vitamin C suboptimal function of vitamin E can also occur. Conversely excessive vitamin E acts as an antagonist for

Table 4.1 Micronutrient function and provisions via PN/EN

Vitamins

Micronutrient	Role/function	At risk groups	Clinical manifestation	Assessment of status (***widely available tests with clinical significance) (**good markers but limited availability) (*little clinical value)	Parenteral nutrition – i.v. supplementation — Vitalipid N†	Parenteral nutrition – i.v. supplementation — Cernevit‡	Enteral nutrition Per 2000 kcal‡
Vitamin A (retinol)	Maintains mucosal integrity and wound healing. Differentiation of tissue	Presence of GI losses and steroid medications	Poor wound healing, impairs neutrophil function	Liver biopsy retinol**. Plasma retinol*	990 µg (3300 µmol)	1050 µg (3500 µmol)	1000–2160 µg
B1 (thiamine)	Decarboxylation in carbohydrate, fat, and alcohol metabolism	Alcoholism. Initiation of high carbohydrate feeding post poor intake "refeeding syndrome"	Refractory metabolic acidosis. Altered neurological state, cardiac effects – wet beri-beri	RBC transketolase***. Blood thiamine**. Urine thiamine or creatinine**	3 mg	3.5 mg	1.4–3.4 mg
B2 (riboflavin)	Oxidative metabolism	Increased requirements as per metabolic rate	Skin/lip lesions, possible impaired immune function	RBC glutathione reductase***. Blood FAD (flavin adenine dinucleotide)**. Urine riboflavin/creatinine***	3.6 mg	4.1 mg	2–6 mg
B3 (niacin)	Active form NAD and NADP in oxidative metabolism	Increased requirements as per metabolic rate	Glossitis with burning in oral cavity – rarely pellagra, diarrhea, dermatitis, dementia	Urine N-methyl nicotinamide**. Blood niacin**	40 mg	46 mg	18–45 mg
B6 (pyridoxine)	Metabolism of amino acids – related to protein requirements. Synthesis of heme and neurotransmitters	CRF – levels decreased in renal failure	Anemia, lesions on skin/lips	RBC transaminase (high activation suggests deficiency)***. Blood pyridoxal *	4.0 mg	4.5 mg	2–13.8 mg
Biotin	Carboxylase reactions – lipogenesis and gluconeogenesis	Non-specified – often in combination with other B vitamin deficiencies	Very rarely as scaly dermatitis, hair loss	Serum biotin**. Urine biotin**	60 µg	69 µg	100–660 µg
Vitamin B12	Coenzyme for conversion of folic acid to active form, valine metabolism	Gastric complications – gastrectomy, congenital intrinsic factor deficiency, malabsorption, IBD, low dietary intake – vegetarians, vegan, and alcoholism	Macrocytic, megablastic anemia, demyelination of neurones	Serum vitamin B12***. Serum homocysteine or cystathionine **	–	6 µg	4.2–6.8 µg
Folate	Active form – tetrahydrofolic acid, role in single carbon transfers: DNA, purine, pyrimidine synthesis	Alcoholism, institutionalized elderly, pregnancy	Macrocytosis, megablastic anemia, neural tube defect in pregnancy	Serum folate***. RBC folate***. Serum homocysteine (often low during supplementation)	400 µg	414 µg	340–880 µg

Micronutrient	Role/function	At risk groups	Clinical manifestation	Assessment of status (***widely available tests with clinical significance) (**good markers but limited availability) (*little clinical value)	Parenteral nutrition – i.v. supplementation		Enteral nutrition Per 2000 kcal†
					Additrace†	Decan‡	
Vitamin C (ascorbic acid)	Antioxidant Absorption of iron	Low socio-economic background pre-admission Requirements secondary to oxidative stress	Scurvy, impaired wound healing	Plasma vit C* Leucocyte vit C*	100 mg	125 mg	100–300 mg
Vitamin D (cholecalciferol)	Ca absorption Differentiation of macrophages	Vitamin D decreases during stress although significance is unknown Pre-hospitalization deficiency secondary to ↓skin synthesis (ethnic minorities, institutionalized elderly)	Impact immune status Osteomalacia and osteoporosis irrelevant in critical care setting	Serum 25-hydroxy vitamin D*** Serum Ca/P/alkaline phosphatase ***	5 μg (200 IU)	5.5 μg (220 IU)	8.5–14.6 μg
Vitamin E (α tocopherols)	Antioxidant of membrane Cofactor for Se	Vitamin E decreases during stress. In septic shock paralleled with increased lipid peroxidation indicative of free radical activity		Plasma tocopherols/ cholesterol***	9.1 mg (10 IU)	10.2 mg (11.2 IU)	20–64 mg
Vitamin K	γ-carboxylation synthesis of coagulation factors	No body stores and limited when bacterial synthesis is disturbed. Deficiency common in TPN void of vitamin K	Bleeding disorders	Prothrombin time*** Plasma phylloquinone**	150 μg	–	100–200 μg

Trace elements

Micronutrient	Role/function	At risk groups	Clinical manifestation	Assessment of status (***widely available tests with clinical significance) (**good markers but limited availability) (*little clinical value)	Parenteral nutrition – i.v. supplementation		Enteral nutrition Per 2000 kcal†
					Additrace†	Decan‡	
Chromium	Insulin activity, lipoprotein metabolism	Unknown – limited evidence	Impaired glucose tolerance, peripheral neuropathy	Plasma Cr** Glucose tolerance *	10 μg (0.2 μmol)	15 μg (0.29 μmol)	30–200 μg
Copper	Essential for enzyme activity; cytochrome oxidase, tyrosinase, superoxide dismutase	Presence of severe malabsorption, malnourished infants, individuals on long-term PN, high zinc supplementation, biliary fistula losses	Hypochromic anemia, neutropenia, arrhythmias	Plasma copper/caeruloplasmin with CRP*** Liver copper**	1.3 mg (20 μmol)	0.48mg (7.6 μmol)	2–3.4 mg
Fluoride	Bone mineralization as calcium flurapatite	Areas of unsupplemented water supplies	Little evidence in critical care – longer term dental caries	Urine excretion*	0.95 mg (50 μmol)	1.45 mg (76 μmol)	2–3 mg
Iodine	Thyroxine and triiodothyronine	Rarely occurs in developed countries	Hypothyroidism in adults Cretinism in infants, goiter	Serum T or TSH***	131 μg (1 μmol)	1.5 μg (0.012 μmol)	120–220 μg
Iron	Hemoglobin Myoglobin Cytochrome system	Low dietary intake Alcoholism Increased losses – GI bleed, post-operative losses Impaired absorption – IBD, celiacs, gastric lymphoma, gastritis	Anemia, impaired immune function, hair loss	Serum ferritin with CRP*** Bone marrow iron** Serum iron/IBC*	1.2 mg (20 μmol)	1.0mg (17.9 μmol)	18–32 mg
Manganese	Present in pyruvate carboxylase, superoxide dismutase, arginase	Deficiency state not confirmed in man, reduced excretion in cholestasis	Weight loss and dermatitis, falls in cholesterol and triglyceride concentrations	Plasma Mn** Whole blood Mn** Mitochondrial superoxide dismutase*	0.3 mg (5 μmol)	0.2 mg (3.6 μmol)	2.4–8 mg

Table 4.1 (cont.)

Trace elements

Micronutrient	Role/function	At risk groups	Clinical manifestation	Assessment of status (***widely available tests with clinical significance) (**good markers but limited availability) (*little clinical value)	Parenteral nutrition – i.v. supplementation		Enteral nutrition Per 2000 kcal‡
					Additrace†	Decan‡	
Molybdenum	Cofactor for aldehyde oxidase, xanthine oxidase and sulfite oxidase	Deficiency rarely described	Can cause headaches, lethargy, coma	Plasma Mo** Urine xanthine**	19 µg (0.2 µmol)	25 µg (0.26 µmol)	74–240 µg
Selenium	Glutathione peroxidase – protection against oxidative damage Thyroxine deiodinase	Deficiency rarely described but can occur in long-term PN	Cardiomyopathy (Keshan disease), skeletal myopathy	Plasma Se*** RBC glutathione peroxidase*** Urine Se** Whole blood Se**	30 µg (0.4 µmol)	70 µg (0.89 µmol)	30–130 µg
Zinc	Required for enzymes of intermediary metabolism and protein synthesis	PN/EN with no provision, increased losses in fistula/diarrhea	Poor wound healing, defective immune function, ageusia, dermatitis	Plasma zinc with albumin and CRP*** Leukocyte zinc** Hair zinc*	6.5 mg (100 µmol)	10.0 mg (153 µmol)	13–36 mg

†Fresenius-Kabi; ‡BaxterHealth Care; ‖Range of tube feeds provided within the UK from Nutricia and Abbott Nutrition.
CRP, C reactive protein.

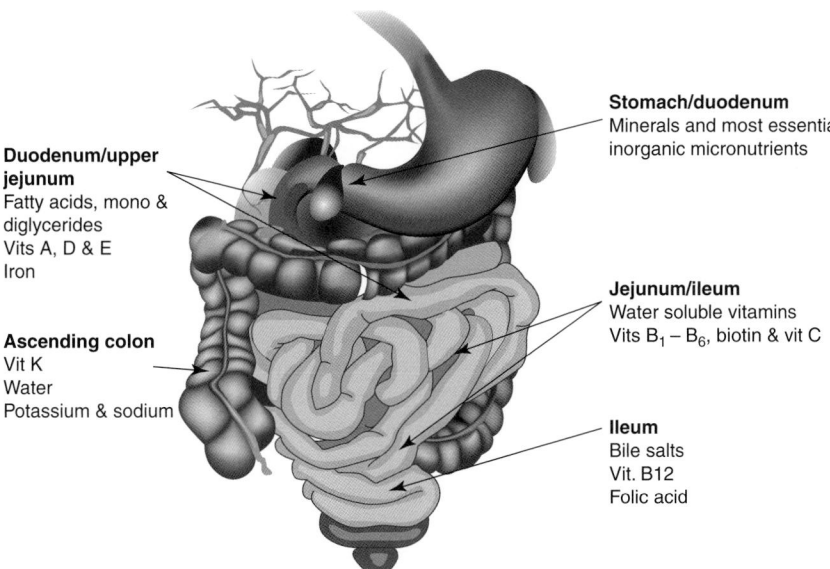

Stomach/duodenum
Minerals and most essential
inorganic micronutrients

Duodenum/upper jejunum
Fatty acids, mono &
diglycerides
Vits A, D & E
Iron

Jejunum/ileum
Water soluble vitamins
Vits B$_1$ – B$_6$, biotin & vit C

Ascending colon
Vit K
Water
Potassium & sodium

Ileum
Bile salts
Vit. B12
Folic acid

Figure 4.1 Sites of absorption of nutrients. (Adapted from The Parenteral and Enteral Nutrition Group of the British Dietetic Association. Pocket Guide to Clinical Nutrition, 3rd ed; 2007: 3.13–3.15.)

vitamin A function. Deficiencies in pyridoxine (B6) and riboflavin (B2) will increase the requirements of niacin (B3). For the aforementioned reasons singular micronutrient supplementation of high doses can also have an adverse impact.

Supplementation of micronutrient vitamins/trace elements in critical care

It is worth noting that in providing EN support, when patients are fed to meet their energy and protein requirements, very often micronutrient and vitamin requirements will be met when using a complete formula. However, total parenteral nutrition (TPN) will not always be complete in terms of vitamins and trace elements and may need to be added within the clinical setting due to storage and stability issues. This requires expert input from specialized nutrition support professionals.

Summary points

Current guidance

- In critically ill or injured patients requiring artificial nutrition full requirements of fluid, electrolytes, vitamins, and minerals should be provided from the outset of feeding.

- PN prescriptions should include "1 daily dose" of multivitamins and trace elements (Grade C).
- Doses of micronutrients in critical care should probably be adapted in proportion to other substrates and severity of underlying disease etiology (Grade C).
- In the presence of major weight variations adaptations of "1 daily dose" should be considered (Grade C).
- Patients on continuous renal replacement therapy or individuals with major burns require additional daily supplementation secondary to continuous effluent losses of water-soluble micronutrients – varying between 1 and 2 extra doses of selenium, zinc, and thiamine on top of the calculated PN requirements (Grade C).
- In ICU patients with possible thiamine deficiency, and especially where alcohol abuse is suspected, commence supplementation of 100–300 mg for the first 3 days to prevent neurological side effects associated with glucose delivery of PN (Grade B).
- A combination of antioxidant vitamins and trace minerals (specifically including selenium) should be provided to all critically ill patients receiving specialized nutrition therapy (Grade B).

Current research

Supplemental antioxidant nutrients: combined vitamins and trace elements
- Antioxidant nutrients, i.e., combined vitamins and trace elements are associated with a significant reduction in mortality in critically ill patients.
- Associated with a trend towards a reduction in hospital length of stay in critically ill patients with significant reduction in ventilator days.
- Evidence suggests no effect on infectious complications in critically ill patients and no effect on ICU length of stay.

Further reading

Ayling R, Marshall W. Nutrition and Laboratory Medicine. London: ACB Venture Publication; 2007.

Berger M, Shenkin A, Revelly JP, et al. Copper, selenium, zinc and thiamine balances during continuous venovenous hemodiafiltration in critically ill patients. Am J Clin Nutr 2004;80:410–416.

Bonet Saris A, Márquez Vácaro JA, Serón Arbeloa C, et al. Guidelines for specialized nutritional and metabolic support in the critically-ill patient. Update. Consensus SEMICYUC-SENPE: Macronutrient and micronutrient requirements. Medicina Intensiva 2011;35 (Suppl 1):17–21.

Critical Care Nutrition, CERU. Practice Guidelines: Supplemental Antioxidant Nutrients: Combined Vitamins and Trace Elements; 2009.

McClave S, Martindale RG, Vanek VW, et al. ASPEN Guidelines for the Provision and Assessment of Nutrition Support Therapy in the Adult Critically Ill Patient. J Parenter Enteral Nutr 2009;33(3):277–316.

NICE and the National Collaborating Centre for Acute Care. Nutrition Support in Adults: Oral Nutrition Support, Enteral Tube Feeding and Parenteral Nutrition. London: NICE and the National Collaborating Centre For Acute Care; 2006.

Shenkin A. Basics in clinical nutrition: Trace elements and vitamins in parenteral and enteral nutrition. ESPEN 2008;3(6):293–297.

Singer P et al. ESPEN Guidelines on Parenteral Nutrition: Intensive Care. Clinical Nutrition (Edinburgh, Scotland). 2009. 28(4):387–400

The Parenteral and Enteral Nutrition Group of the British Dietetic Association. Pocket Guide to Clinical Nutrition, 3rd edn London: PEN Group Publications; 2007;3.13–3.15.

Ziegler T. Parenteral nutrition in the critically ill patient. New Engl J Med 2009;361 (11):1088–1097.

5

Enteral and parenteral feeding protocols

Malissa Warren and Robert Martindale

Introduction

Nutritional support has traditionally been regarded as a means to provide basic energy for cellular homeostasis while amino acids are considered necessary for protein synthesis. However, patients admitted to intensive care units are in a dynamic state between systemic inflammation, immune suppression, and persistent chronic inflammatory states. It often takes weeks or months for the inflammatory states resulting from ICU admission to resolve. Multiple factors including timing of insult, pre-stress co-morbidities will influence the duration of the hyperdynamic inflammatory state. The ability to attenuate the metabolic response to stress has recently been proven in most ICU populations. Obtaining the maximal benefit from this metabolic modulation requires rapid and rather specific nutrient delivery. Evidence suggests that feeding protocols improve the delivery of nutrition to critically ill patients by promoting early initiation and enhanced adequacy of EN. Globally at least six major nutrition societies have published critical care nutrition guidelines over the past 15 years providing some consensus in areas of critical care nutrition. However, worldwide agreement among professional organizations exists for the preference of early enteral nutrition compared to parenteral nutrition in the critically ill patient. Unfortunately, recent multinational, observational studies demonstrate a significant gap between our knowledge and the application of evidence-based nutrition practices. This reveals the complexity of the critical care setting where nutrition therapy varies around the world in different patient populations and diverse intensive care unit (ICU) cultures. This abundance and sometimes discrepancy of information creates confusion and skepticism for the critical care provider who is attempting to apply evidence-based critical care nutrition guidelines. Protocols have become the foundation for hospitals to translate evidenced-based guidelines into bedside application. Protocols can guide a complex decision-making process, closing gaps in knowledge and practice, optimizing the quality of patient care, and promoting cost effectiveness.

Nutrition in Critical Care, ed. Peter Faber and Mario Siervo. Published by Cambridge University Press. © Cambridge University Press 2014.

Importance of feeding protocols

Since the 1950s the literature demonstrates that 30 to 50% of hospitalized patients remain malnourished. In addition, at least a third of patients experience significant deterioration in their nutritional status during hospitalization. Critically ill patients are at significant risk for iatrogenic malnutrition due to the obligatory catabolic effects of the severity of illness and the lack of or delayed feeding common in the ICU setting. It is well-supported in the critical care literature that malnourished patients suffer more infections, exhibit poor wound healing, spend more time on the ventilators, have extended length of both ICU stay and hospital stay, and have increased risk of mortality compared to their nourished counterparts. Though it is often difficult to determine the optimal quantity of nutrition in critically ill patients, recent studies demonstrate that a deficit of as little as 10 000 kcal in the first week can result in prolonged mechanical ventilation, increased risk of pneumonia, and prolonged hospital stays. Previous work showed that patients in the ICU received 51.6% of goal EN volume throughout their ICU stay and caloric deficits greater than 12 000 calories were observed during the first week of ICU care, which correlated with increased infectious complications. Unfortunately, attempting to compensate for deficits occurring in the first week was not associated with reduced complications. In 2008, Faisy et al. conducted an observational study of ICU patients requiring prolonged mechanical ventilation and revealed that a negative energy balance in the first 14 days in the ICU was an independent factor of mortality. Another large multicenter multinational observational study reported a reduction in mortality and ventilator-free days for every 1000 calorie increase in energy provision and additional 30 g in protein provision, particularly for patients at the extremes of BMI. Thus the primary goals of feeding protocols are to synthesize evidence-based guidelines for best nutrition practice and improve the provision of early enteral feeding in the ICU, reduce morbidity and mortality, and decrease malnutrition-associated hospital costs.

Review of the evidence for enteral and parenteral feeding protocols

Many before and after studies have evaluated the impact of feeding protocols on nutrition practice in the ICU and consistently demonstrate that feeding protocols are associated with increased use and/or infusion of EN. Table 5.1 provides a summary of recent studies and their feeding protocols for reference. Some of these studies are described further.

Taylor and colleagues performed a prospective, randomized, controlled trial in mechanically ventilated patients following head injury to determine the effect of early enhanced enteral nutrition on clinical outcomes. EN was initiated at goal rate

Table 5.1 Summary of studies and protocols

Protocol	Patient population	Protocol features
Spain et al. (1999)	Medical	Early EN
		Avoidance of holding EN for diagnostic tests, routine nursing care, or bedside procedures
Kozar et al. (2002)	Trauma, TBI (traumatic brain injury), surgical	Early EN
		Management of tolerance to EN
Taylor et al. (1999)	Trauma, TBI	Early EN starting at goal rate versus titration over time
Martin et al. (2004) ACCEPT Trial	Medical, surgical	Management of diarrhea with EN
		Assessment of tolerance to EN
Doig et al. (2008)	Medical, surgical	Early EN
		Management of diarrhea with EN
Pousman et al. (2009)	Surgical	Decreased pre-operative fasting
Heyland et al. (2010) PEP uP Protocol	Medical, surgical	24-hour volume-based feeding goals to maximize EN delivery. Nurse-driven algorithm to increase infusion rate in order to account for interruptions
Singer et al. (2011)	Medical, surgical	Repeated indirect calorimetry measurements and supplemental PN to cover calorie shortfalls delivered by EN
Miller et al. (2011)	Medical, surgical, trauma	Integrates evaluation of severity of illness with nutrition assessment and therapy plan
Soguel et al. (2012)	Medical, surgical	Bottom-up protocol
		Supplemental PN added by day 4 if EN provides less than 60% of estimated needs
		Dedicated ICU dietitian

in the intervention group versus titrating from 15 ml/hour over time in the control group. By starting EN at goal infusion rate, the intervention group received almost twice the percentage of goal calories compared to the control group and had a significantly lower incidence of infectious complications, 61% versus 85% in controls. Patients in the intervention group also demonstrated a trend toward enhanced neurological recovery at 3 months.

In a prospective study of patients with major trauma, Kozar et al. established the success of a standardized enteral protocol focusing on the management of intolerance to EN. The protocol provided specific guidance in the event of vomiting, abdominal distention, diarrhea, high nasogastric (NG) output, and medication contraindications with feeding such as inotropic agents and paralytics. The majority of patients managed by the standardized protocol exhibited tolerance as defined by EN advancement per protocol with few patients requiring reduction in EN infusion rate or holding of EN feeding. Evaluating the value of nutrition protocols in increasing nutrient delivery Spain et al. showed improved EN delivery in following implementation of a nutrition protocol. This implementation reported a 30% increase in patients receiving more than 90% of goal EN. Mackenzie and colleagues also showed that implementation of an evidence-based feeding protocol improved EN delivery from 20% before implementing the feeding protocol to 80% post-protocol implementation. In addition PN use was reduced in the post implementation group. In a similar prospective before and after protocol implementation study, Barr et al. also demonstrated that implementation of a feeding protocol that initiated feeding within 48 hours of admission was associated with more patients receiving EN. Clinical outcomes of this study included shortened duration of mechanical ventilation and a reduction in mortality associated with EN protocol utilization in the study patients.

In a recent international prospective observational cohort study the effect of enteral feeding protocols was evaluated in nearly 6000 patients. Hospitals utilizing evidence-based feeding protocols used more EN, started EN approximately 16 hours earlier, and used more prokinetic agents in cases of elevated gastric residual volumes compared with sites that did not use a feeding protocol. Overall nutritional adequacy and intake from EN were higher at protocol sites versus non-protocol sites.

In a large Australian study, Doig et al. evaluated whether nutritional guidelines can improve ICU feeding practices and reduce mortality in ICU patients. In this cluster randomized controlled trial (RCT), ICUs following guidelines fed patients earlier and achieved caloric goals more often. However, hospital mortality, the primary outcome of the study, was not different between the guideline and control ICUs. Control ICUs were initiating EN in 1.37 days versus 0.75 days at study sites. Clearly, both sites were meeting guideline recommendations for early feeding practices thus lack of a mortality difference is not unexpected.

Elements of feeding protocols

To allow optimal incorporation and timely initiation, feeding protocols should be incorporated into the ICU admission orders. Feeding protocols enable the bedside nurse and ICU team to initiate and improve the delivery of EN in a timely manner without prolonged delay that may occur in the ICU setting. Protocols may be preprinted order sets or algorithms or computerized templates. Figures 5.1 and 5.2 provide examples of preprinted algorithm and computerized templates for feeding protocols.

The elements of feeding protocols vary; though common topics include guidance for the timing of feeding, route of feeding (EN versus PN), selection of feeding formula (immune-enhancing versus standard EN formula), titration schedules, strategies for optimizing administration such as modifications in treatment for elevated gastric residuals or minimizing time patients spend NPO. In addition, protocols describe strategies to reduce risks of feeding such as aspiration, over- or underfeeding, and poor glycemic control. Table 5.2

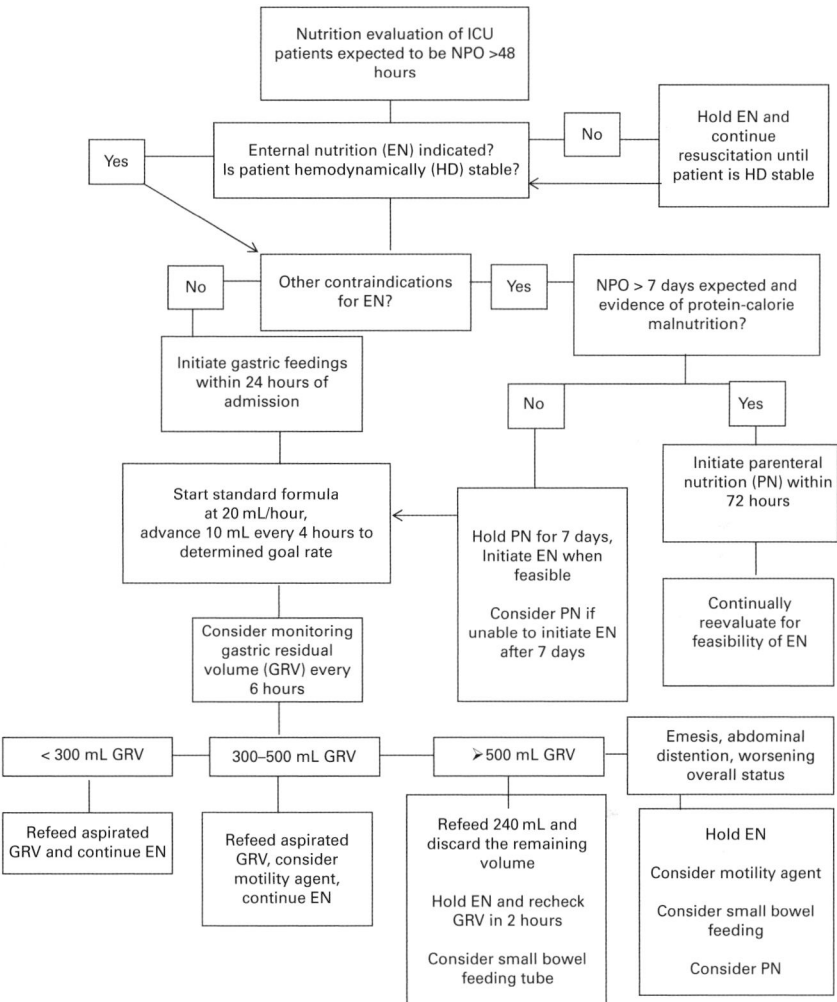

Figure 5.1 Sample critical care nutrition feeding algorithm.

provides some common elements of feeding protocols as well as specific examples from written feeding protocols.

Developing and implementing a feeding protocol

Common obstacles to early nutrient delivery contributing to delay in enteral feeding in the ICU include under-prescribing of EN by critical care providers, slow titration, and frequent interruptions of EN for a variety of laboratory and radiological procedures and even routine nursing care such as bathing, changing linens. Many

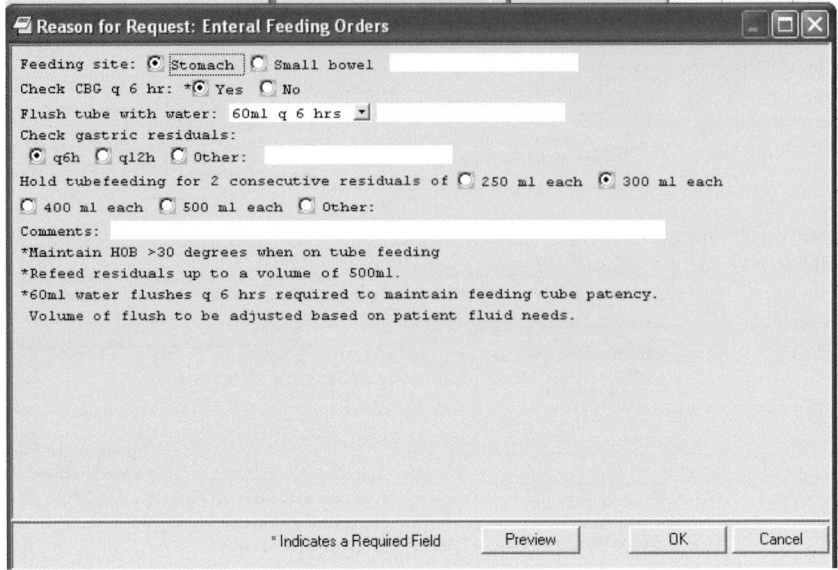

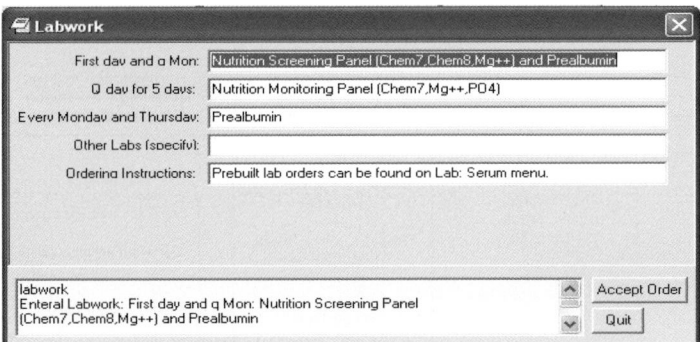

Figure 5.2 Sample templates from a computerized enteral feeding protocol.

of the obstacles may stem from a lack of ICU team education on the importance of nutrition in the ICU setting. Several recent surveys of ICU physicians indicate a significant lack of knowledge regarding evidence-based nutrition guidelines. Moreover, ICU physicians and nurses are focusing on multiple evidence-based protocols or tasks that they may see as a priority to nutrition care in the ICU. These obstacles commonly lead to a lack of compliance with feeding protocols by critical care clinicians, limiting protocol effectiveness. Spain et al. measured a 42% protocol non-compliance rate by critical care providers in their study described previously. Barr and colleagues illustrated similar problems with protocol adherence. The suggestion that the team involved in bedside implementation should have

Table 5.2 Common elements of feeding protocols

Elements of critical care nutrition feeding protocols	Examples
Timing of enteral nutrition	Initiate EN within 24 hours of admission to ICU or when patient has completed resuscitation phase of ICU stay
Enteral formula selection Standard versus specialized formulas Fiber versus non-fiber-containing formulas	Immune-enhancing or metabolic modulating formulations indicated in post-operative GI cancer surgery and trauma
Titration of enteral nutrition	Initiate at 20 mL/hour then advance 20 mL every 6 hours based on tolerance
Monitoring of enteral nutrition	Refeed GRVs (gastric residual volumes) < 500 mL and continue EN delivery. Monitor closely for other signs of intolerance such as abdominal distention and/or pain, hypotension, nausea/vomiting Consider prokinetic if GRVs > 300–500 mL for two consecutive checks Maintain glycemic control 5.5–10.0 mmol/L
Guidance for optimizing enteral nutrition delivery	If EN is interrupted, increase infusion rate to make up for missed EN volume to achieve the daily goal volume If feeding distal to the stomach, hold EN for no more than 2 hours prior to surgery Do not stop EN for diagnostic tests or standard nursing care
Timing of parenteral nutrition	Avoid PN for first week of ICU stay in previously well-nourished patients
Parenteral nutrition prescription	Avoid use of soybean oil-based lipid emulsion in first week of ICU stay Use conservative calorie prescription such as 20 kcal/kg estimated dry body weight
Monitoring of parenteral nutrition	Maintain glycemic control 5.5–10.0 mmol/L Monitor appropriate labs daily

direct ongoing involvement in protocol improvement has proven successful in a variety of ICUs. Protocol compliance and performance should be routinely assessed and measured with timely feedback directly to the clinicians utilizing the protocol. Doig et al. achieved significant practice change with an extensive guideline implementation strategy in their cluster randomized study. Guideline implementation consisted of a 2-day guideline development conference with an educational workshop on the use of the multi-faceted change strategy. The change strategy included identification of opinion leaders, education outreach visits for guideline initiation, academic detailing in order to provide evidence or information to clinicians who are reluctant to adopt guidelines, active reminders (dietitian reviewing ICU patients twice daily and discussing those who qualified for the guideline with senior staff), timely audit and feedback, passive reminders (posters, algorithms posted around the ICU), and in-servicing. In a prospective interventional study evaluating methods of protocol implementation, Soguel and colleagues identified nine major areas for evidence-based practice improvement. The group then developed a bottom-up protocol using an interdisciplinary team to build reference materials for training on the protocol implementation. As part of a multiphase trial all clinicians working in the ICU received a copy of the feeding protocol. Two dietitians provided regular education to each ICU clinician upon implementation and regular education sessions were introduced into the routine ICU education program as well as an introduction for new staff orientation. During the last phase of the study, a dedicated and knowledgeable ICU dietitian was present in order to advise other ICU team members as needed about the protocol. The combined intervention of the ongoing evidence-based feeding protocol and the presence of a dedicated ICU dietitian improved caloric delivery by 31.6%.

Implementing successful feeding protocols requires an astute multi-disciplinary group who is prepared to review the weaknesses in their current bedside nutrition practice and consider consensus guidelines that would be most relevant to improve nutrition therapy in their ICU. Recommendations associated with feeding protocols should be easily interpreted, cost effective, and have the ability to be implemented with available resources. As noted earlier protocol compliance can limit the effectiveness of feeding protocols. In order to overcome resistance to protocol compliance, stakeholders should be identified and given the opportunity to provide ongoing feedback for implementation and revision of the protocol. Also the protocol performance and adherence must be routinely assessed with direct feedback to the individuals implementing the protocols. As previously mentioned above feedback through audits and benchmarking reports on performance of key elements in critical care nutrition guidelines significantly improved the use and adequacy of EN and PN when appropriate.

Because protocols and guidelines do not account for all circumstances in an intensive care setting, a provider's clinical judgment remains essential to patient care and will of course override any protocol if concern for patient safety is in question.

Summary points

- Even a small negative energy balance results in prolonged mechanical ventilation and hospital stay.
- In mechanically ventilated patients a negative energy balance is a predictor of mortality.
- Early goal-directed feeding protocols improve calorie intake in critical care patients.
- Implementation of feeding protocols involve critical care physicians, nurses, and dietitians.

Further reading

Barr J, Hecht M, Flavin K, et al. Outcomes in critically ill patients before and after the implementation of an evidence-based nutritional management protocol. Chest 2004;125:1446–1457.

Doig G, Simpson F, Finfer S, et al. Effect of evidence-based feeding guidelines on mortality of critically ill adults. A cluster randomized controlled trial. JAMA 2008;300:2731–2741.

Faisy C, Lerolle N, Dachraoui F, et al. Impact of energy deficit calculated by a predictive method on outcome in medical patients requiring prolonged acute mechanical ventilation. Br J Nutr 2009;101:1079–1087.

Heyland D, Cahill N, Dhaliwal R, et al. Impact of enteral feeding protocols on enteral nutrition delivery: results of a multicenter observational study. J Parenter Enteral Nutr 2010;34:675–684.

Kozar R, McQuiggan M, Moore E, et al. Postinjury enteral tolerance is reliably achieved by a standardized protocol. J Surg Res 2002;104:70–75.

Mackenzie S, Zygun D, Whitmore B, et al. Implementation of a nutrition support protocol increases the proportion of mechanically ventilated patients reaching enteral nutrition targets in the adult intensive care unit. J Parenter Enteral Nutr 2005;29:74–80.

Martin C, Doig G, Heyland D, et al. Multicentre, cluster-randomized clinical trial of algorithms for critical-care enteral and parenteral therapy. Can Med Assoc J 2004;170:197–204.

Miller KR, Kiraly LN, Lowen CC, Martindale RG, McClave SA. "CAN WE FEED?" A mnemonic to merge nutrition and intensive care assessment of the critically ill patient. J Parenter Enteral Nutr. 2011;35(5):643–659.

Pousman RM, Pepper C, Pandharipande P, et al. Feasibility of implementing a reduced fasting protocol for critically ill trauma patients undergoing operative and nonoperative procedures. J Parenter Enteral Nutr 2009;33(2):176–180.

Singer P, Anbar R, Cohen J, et al. The tight calorie control study (TICACOS): a prospective, randomized, controlled pilot study of nutritional support in critically ill patients. Intensive Care Med 2011;37(4):601–609.

Spain D, McClave S, Sexton L, et al. Infusion protocol improves delivery of enteral tube feeding in the critical care unit. J Parenter Enteral Nutr 1999;23:288–292.

Soguel L, Revelly JP, Schaller MD, et al. Energy deficit and length of hospital stay can be reduced by a two-step quality improvement of nutrition therapy: the intensive care unit dietitian can make the difference. Crit Care Med 2012;40:412–419.

Taylor S, Fettes S, Jewkes C, et al. Prospective, randomized, controlled trial to determine the effect of early enhanced enteral nutrition on clinical outcome of head-injured patients. Crit Care Med 1999;27:2525–2531.

6

Commercial nutritional enteral and parenteral formulations in critical care

Jonathan A. Silversides, Stephen T. Webb, and Andrew J. Ferguson

Introduction

The clinician tasked with procurement or prescribing of nutritional support for the critically ill patient is faced with a wide and dynamic range of products that can appear bewildering. A sound understanding of the basic components and properties of these products will facilitate informed decision-making and allow for a rational assessment of new products as they appear. It is not possible to provide a detailed analysis of all available products, and we have provided details on a sample from the most widely used enteral and parenteral formulas in the United Kingdom at present. We recommend obtaining up to date information from the manufacturer before prescribing any form of nutritional support.

Enteral nutrition formulas

Enteral nutrition formulas typically contain varying proportions of carbohydrate, fat, and nitrogen (in the form of protein, peptides, or amino acids), together with electrolytes, trace elements, and vitamins. Enteral nutrition is generally presented as a fluid/liquid formulation. The formulation may contain specific immuno-modulating nutrients or fiber.

Total energy intake

Energy requirements in the critically ill patient are highly variable, depending on body habitus, baseline nutritional state, acute illness, and degree of activity. Current guidelines from the European Society for Clinical Nutrition and Metabolism (ESPEN) recommend a total energy intake of 20–25 kCal/kg/day for critically ill patients, which is typically provided as a combination of protein,

Nutrition in Critical Care, ed. Peter Faber and Mario Siervo. Published by Cambridge University Press. © Cambridge University Press 2014.

carbohydrate, and lipid. This may be increased in those with severe malnutrition and during the anabolic recovery phase to a maximum of 30 kCal/kg/day.

Protein and amino acids

Proteins, peptides, or amino acids account for 15–25% of the energy provision in most formulas, with the rest made up of variable proportions of carbohydrate and lipid. In order to achieve adequate protein intake of 1.2–1.5 g/kg/day, and prevent excessive catabolism and loss of muscle mass, formulas providing a higher percentage of calories as protein are preferable.

Protein is generally provided as intact soy, whey, or casein polypeptide chains containing essential and non-essential amino acids. Whey protein is rich in cysteine, and has been postulated to promote production of glutathione, an antioxidant, and thus to have an anti-inflammatory effect, although this remains unsubstantiated to date.

For patients at risk of malabsorption, enteral feeds containing only single free amino acids, or di- and tripeptides, have been developed, usually along with fatty acids and oligosaccharides. These are known as elemental or semi-elemental formulas. While these formulas have an established role in inflammatory bowel disease, particularly in children, it is in the setting of acute pancreatitis that they are of most interest in critical care. By reducing digestive requirements, it is postulated that secretion of destructive pancreatic enzymes may be reduced. This approach is considerably more expensive, and so far has not been demonstrated to offer any significant benefit over standard polymeric formulas.

There has also been considerable interest in the role of essential branched-chain amino acids (leucine, isoleucine, and valine) in chronic liver disease, following the observation that these are deficient in many cirrhotic patients and that deficiency of isoleucine in particular is associated with hepatic encephalopathy. Enteral formulas enriched in these branched-chain amino acids are available, are associated with minor cognitive improvements in hepatic encephalopathy, and may be beneficial in reducing the catabolic state that exists in patients with cirrhosis.

Carbohydrate

The carbohydrate component of enteral formulas is usually provided in the form of hydrolyzed starches such as maltodextrin, although formulas designed for oral (as opposed to gastric or post-gastric) use will contain some oligosaccharides such as sucrose to improve palatability. Almost all are lactose-free. Concerns regarding excessive carbohydrate content relate to hyperglycemia, hyperlipidemia, hepatic dysfunction, and increased carbon dioxide generation.

Fat

Fats represent an efficient energy source, with 9 kCal/g compared with 4 kCal/g for carbohydrates and proteins. Higher fat:carbohydrate ratios are therefore often used in concentrated feeds. Traditional lipid sources such as soy and corn oil contain mainly long-chain fatty acids and these require bile salts and lipases for emulsification and digestion. For this reason many feeds, particularly those designed for patients with malabsorption, contain medium-chain fatty acids, derived from coconut oil and other sources, which can be absorbed directly into the portal system even in the setting of biliary or pancreatic dysfunction. The lower respiratory quotient for most fats compared with carbohydrate leads to a theoretical advantage of lower carbon dioxide production in patients fed with higher fat formulas, but this has not been shown to translate into clinically meaningful outcome benefits.

Other important features of lipid content include the proportion of omega (ω)-6 (derived mainly from sunflower, safflower, soy, and corn oils) and ω-3- fatty acids (derived mainly from fish oils). ω-6-fatty acids such as linoleic acid are precursors of arachidonic acid and pro-inflammatory prostaglandins and leukotrienes. The conditionally essential ω-6 fatty acid gamma-linolenic acid (GLA) and ω-3-fatty acids such as α-linolenic acid (ALA) and eicosapentaenoic acid (EPA) are involved in production of anti-inflammatory mediators such as Prostaglandin E_1, and supplementation of these has been the subject of considerable interest in acute respiratory distress syndrome and sepsis. Despite promising results in early studies in acute lung injury, the largest and most recent trial was recently stopped early for futility and a possibility of harm.

Fiber

Standard enteral feeds do not usually contain fiber. However, fiber-containing versions of most formulas are available, and are often used in an attempt to reduce or prevent enteral feeding-associated diarrhea. The role of fiber is incompletely understood. It is postulated that specific soluble fibers such as inulins and fructo-oligosaccharides may act as a fermentable substrate for normal gut flora, inhibiting overgrowth of pathogenic bacteria and promoting production of short-chain fatty acids such as butyrate, the major energy source for colonic mucosa. This may, in turn, improve mucosal barrier function and improve absorption of sodium and water, reducing diarrhea. Conversely, the increased peristalsis and reduced gut transit time may worsen absorption and exacerbate diarrhea.

The results of a few small studies suggest that the use of feeds containing soluble fiber may reduce the incidence of diarrhea in critically ill patients, although this is not yet established, and its effectiveness may be limited by the use of broad-spectrum antibiotics. Insoluble fiber, on the other hand, has not been shown to be of benefit, and intestinal obstruction has been reported as a complication of its use in patients with decreased bowel motility.

Immunonutrition

Arginine is regarded as a conditionally essential amino acid which is involved in lymphocyte function and connective tissue repair and which is a precursor of nitric oxide production. Deficiency of arginine is common in the critically ill, and arginine supplementation has been extensively studied in a variety of populations.

Arginine supplementation is associated with no benefit in a general ICU population and a possible increase in mortality in the most severely ill patients (APACHE II score >25), postulated to be due to increased nitric oxide production and vasodilation. In elective surgical patients, however, both pre- and post-operative supplementation of arginine is associated with a marked reduction in infectious complications, improved wound healing, and shorter length of stay. This effect appears consistent in subpopulations undergoing gastrointestinal, head and neck, and cardiac surgery with both pre- and post-operative administration.

Glutamine is the most abundant amino acid in the body. It also has the highest flux rate and hence glutamine is rapidly depleted in critical illness, and is therefore regarded as conditionally essential. Among other functions, glutamine is a major metabolic substrate for enterocytes, leukocytes, and other cells with rapid turnover, and may therefore have an important role in gut mucosal integrity and immune function. Studies examining glutamine supplementation have reported a reduction in the rate of infectious complications and in hospital length of stay in critically ill patients with trauma and burns; with a reduction in mortality only in patients with burns. However, larger and more recent trials reported no benefit and evidence of increased mortality in a general ICU population.

Micronutrients

There has been considerable interest in the role of antioxidant vitamins and minerals, particularly selenium, as therapeutic agents in the critically ill. In a recent meta-analysis, replacement of micronutrients in quantities greater than routinely given as part of enteral or parenteral nutrition is associated with decreased mortality in ICU patients. The studies included in the meta-analysis were heterogeneous and it is far from clear which micronutrient or combination of micronutrients, and by which delivery route, may be beneficial. Antioxidant supplementation was associated with no benefit in a recent large randomized controlled trial and remains unsupported by available evidence.

Current guidelines support the administration of sufficient quantities of vitamins and minerals to prevent deficiencies. All commercially available formulas contain sufficient concentrations of vitamins, micronutrients, and trace elements to meet recommended daily intake when absorbed in sufficient quantities to meet macronutrient needs. There is therefore little to choose between the various formulas on the basis of vitamin or micronutrient content. Consideration should be given to specific supplementation of vitamins and minerals in patients who are not absorbing full rate enteral feeds. This is particularly important in those patients with additional micronutrient losses during continuous renal replacement therapy.

Nucleotides

Nucleotides are the components of DNA, RNA, and ATP, and are essential for cellular proliferation. Accordingly, an adequate supply of nucleotides is most important for rapidly dividing cells such as lymphocytes and enterocytes, and administration of nucleotides by the parenteral or enteral route has been associated with improved intestinal mucosal integrity, decreased bacterial translocation, and improved immune function in animal models of sepsis. Although it remains uncertain whether this translates into meaningful clinical benefit in humans, nucleotides have been incorporated into some enteral formulas.

Low volume formulas and osmolality

Concentrated feeds are available for patients who require fluid restriction, for example heart failure or anuric renal failure patients. While standard concentration feeds contain 1 to 1.25 kCal/mL, low volume feeds contain between 1.5 and 2 kCal/mL. However, due to the relative insolubility of protein, it is difficult to meet protein needs using these formulas, and since these groups of patients are particularly catabolic, it is essential that protein intake is adequate. In the ICU setting any excessive volume load from feeds can usually be managed by titrated use of diuretics or by ultrafiltration, without recourse to more concentrated formulas. Formulas with 1.25 to 1.5 kCal/mL may assist with calorie and nutrient provision during establishment of enteral feeding where intake volumes are lower, although osmolality and tolerance may have to be taken into account.

The osmolality of an enteral formula is determined by the quantities of oligo- and di-saccharides, amino acids and nucleotides, as well as soluble fibers such as inulin. It has been postulated that use of formulas with higher osmolality may cause movement of free water into the gut lumen, contributing to rapid gut transit and osmotic diarrhea. The occurrence of diarrhea appears to be more related to the quantity of fermentable oligo-, di-, and mono-saccharides (FODMAPs) than to osmolality, and this cannot be predicted from the published ingredients. In short, there is no evidence that the osmolality of a formula has any significant impact on tolerance or side effects of enteral nutrition (Table 6.1).

Selecting the right enteral nutrition formula for your patient

For the majority of general ICU patients, there is generally little evidence on which to base decisions regarding the choice of one enteral formula over another. Any of the "standard" enteral formulas, if given in adequate quantities, will meet the nutritional needs of most ICU patients. This is reassuring since choices are often made on economic and practical grounds and perhaps as the result of procurement and tendering processes across multiple hospitals.

For certain patient groups, however, there is evidence that the addition of immune-modulating nutrients can influence outcome. For example, trauma patients appear to benefit from glutamine supplementation, which may be given as part of an immune-enhancing formula, e.g., Impact with Glutamine®, or separately as an intravenous or enteral supplement.

Table 6.1 Components of selected enteral tube feeding formulations (all components are presented per 1000 mL).

Manufacturer	Brand	% Energy as: kcal	N$_2$	Fat	Carbohydrate	N$_2$ source	Fat source	Carbohydrate source	Fibre (g)	Osmolality (mOsmol/kg)	Linolenic acid (g)	Linoleic acid (g)	Na+ (mmol)	Glutamine (g)	Arginine (g)
Standard formulas															
Nutricia	Nutrison	1000	16	35	49	Milk protein	Vegetable oils	Maltodextrin	<1	265	–	–	43	–	0
Fresenius Kabi	Fresubin Original	1000	15	30	55	Milk, soy protein	Rapeseed, sunflower, fish oil	Maltodextrin, sucrose	0.1	250	2.1	8.5	33	0.3	0
Abbott	Jevity	1100	15	29	53	Casein	Sunflower, canola, Corn oil, MCTs, vegetable oil	Maltodextrin	17.6	300	0.9	6.2	40.4	3.9	1.4
Nestle	Novasource GI Control	1100	15	28	53	Milk protein	Vegetable oils	Maltodextrin	21	286	–	–	30.4	–	–
Fresenius Kabi	Fresubin 1000	1000	22	24	50	Milk protein	Rapeseed, sunflower, fish oil	Maltodextrin	2	360	2.3	5.6	67	5.2	20
Nutricia	Nutrison Low Sodium	1000	16	35	49	Milk protein	Vegetable oils	Maltodextrin	0	240	–	–	11	–	–
Abbott	Jevity Plus HP	1300	25	30	43	Milk, soy protein	Sunflower, canola, MCT, corn oils	Maltodextrin	15	385	1.2	4.4	43.5	8.3	3.1
Abbott	Osmolite	1000	16	30	54	Milk, soy protein	Sunflower, canola, MCT oils	Maltodextrin	0	288	1	3.9	38.3	3.9	1.6
Nutricia	Nutrison MCT	1000	20	30	50	Milk protein	60% MCT, vegetable oils	Maltodextrin	0	315	–	–	43	–	–
Concentrated (low volume) formulas															
Abbott	TwoCal	2000	17	40	42	Milk protein	Sunflower, canola, soy	Corn syrup, maltodextrin	10	800	2.1	19.3	56.5	9.1	2.8
Nutricia	Nutrison Concentrated	2000	15	45	40	Milk protein	Vegetable oils	Maltodextrin	0	470	–	–	43	–	–
Fresenius Kabi	Fresubin HP Energy	1500	20	35	45	Milk protein	MCT, vegetable oils, fish oils	Maltodextrin	0	400	2.4	11.8	52	7.2	2.8

Fresenius Kabi	Fresenius 2250	1500	15	35	48	Milk and soy protein	Vegetable, fish oils	Maltodextrin	15	430	4.2	11	43	5.2	3.4
Abbott	Nepro	2000	14	43	41	Caseinates	Sunflower, canola oil	Maltodextrin, sucrose	15.6	637	3.1	12.8	36.7	7.1	2.3
Abbott	Jevity 1.5	1500	17	29	52	Milk protein	Sunflower, canola, corn oil, MCTs, vegetable oil	Maltodextrin	22	524	1.4	5.2	60.9	6.2	2.6
Abbott	Osmolite 1.5	1500	17	29	54	Milk, soy protein	Sunflower, canola, MCT oils	Maltodextrin	0	510	1.4	5.3	60.9	6.1	2.5

Elemental and semi-elemental formulas

Nestle	Peptamen	1000	16	33	51	Hydrolysed whey protein	75% MCT	Maltodextrin, modified corn starch	0	270		3.7	24.3		0.9
Nestle	Peptamen ProBio	1000	16	33	51	Hydrolysed whey protein	70% MCT	Maltodextrin, cornstarch	4	300			24.3		
Nutricia	Nutrison Peptisorb	1000	16	15	69	Hydrolysed whey protein	MCT, vegetable oils	Maltodextrin, starch	0	535	–	–	43	–	–
Fresenius Kabi	Suvimed OPD	1000	18	25	57	Hydrolysed whey protein	MCT, vegetable oils	Maltodextrin	0.8	350	0.8	4.5	35	4	0.9
Fresenius Kabi	Reconvan	1000	22	30	48	Hydrolysed wheat protein, arginine	57% MCT, fish oils	Maltodextrin	0	320	0.7	6.9	60	10.2	6.7
Abbott	Perative	1300	20	25	54	Hydrolysed caseinate and whey protein	MCT 40%, canola, corn oils	Maltodextrin	0	385	1.4	6.6	45.2	5.5	8.7
Abbott	Prosure	1270	21	18	58	Partially hydrolysed caseinates, whey protein	Fish oil, MCT, canola, soy oils	Maltodextrin, sucrose	21	599	0.5	1.8	65.2	6.5	2.2

Special purpose formulas

Abbot	Oxepa	1500	17	56	28	Protein	25% MCT	Maltodextrin	0	490	7.1	14	57	6.1	2.1
Nestle	Impact	1000	22	25	53	Casein, arginine	Fish oil, 3.3 g n-FA	Maltodextrin	0	350			47	6.1	13
Abbott	Pulmocare	1500	17	56	28	Casein	Canola, MCT, corn, sunflower oils	Maltodextrin, sucrose	0	488	4.9	19.1	57	6.1	2.1
Fresenius Kabi	Supportan	1500	27	40	33	Milk protein	MCT, fish oils	Maltodextrin, sucrose	12	435	0.2	9.5	21	7.4	3.6
Nestle	Impact with Glutamine	1300	24	30	46	Casein, arginine	MCTs – palm & sunflower oils	Maltodextrin	0	630	3.78 (omega-6)	2.4 (omega-3)	57	15	16.3

For elective peri-operative patients without septic or SIRS (systemic inflammatory response syndrome) shock, arginine supplementation is of benefit in the pre- and early post-operative phase, and may be given in an enteral formula, e.g., Impact®, or as a separate nutritional supplement.

Use of omega-3 fatty acid supplementation is recommended for patients with acute lung injury in current European and North American guidelines. However, these guidelines were published before the most recent (negative) trial, and it would seem that attempts to down-regulate inflammation by this means, although logical, may not be clinically beneficial. For this reason, clinicians may be called upon to justify any additional expenditure required for the provision of formulas such as Oxepa® (Abbot), Impact® (Nestle Nutrition), and Supportan® (Fresenius Kabi) over and above the costs and benefits of standard products. Impact® may, however, still be useful for its high arginine content in selected post-operative patients.

While elemental and semi-elemental feeds do not appear to offer any benefit when used routinely, their use may be considered for those with evidence of, or at high risk for malabsorption, such as those with acute pancreatitis. As well as containing nitrogen as free amino acids or oligo-peptides, in most of these formulas the predominant source of lipid is medium-chain triglycerides, which may improve absorption.

For patients who develop diarrhea while being fed by the enteral route, the primary approach is to exclude serious inflammatory and infectious causes, particularly *Clostridium difficile* colitis. Once this has been done, an empirical trial of a low-osmolality fiber-containing formula is reasonable, although the success of this approach in improving diarrhea, particularly in the context of broad-spectrum antibiotic use, is likely to be limited.

Parenteral nutrition formulas

Parenteral nutrition may be used as the sole form of nutritional support (total parenteral nutrition or TPN), or to supplement enteral feeding during establishment or in cases of poor tolerance and absorption of EN. Disadvantages attributed to the parenteral route include increased infection rates, decreased gut mucosal integrity, and the need for central venous access for most formulas, and there is consensus that the enteral route should be used where possible for nutrition support. Parenteral formulas are available as nutritionally complete packs, but are commonly provided as individual components (e.g., lipid emulsions, glucose and amino acid solutions, multivitamins, etc.) for custom formulation under sterile conditions in hospital pharmacies. This provides great flexibility to specifically tailor support to individual patient needs. Due to instability in storage, complete packs are provided as individual pouches which are mixed immediately prior to being administered to the patient. Once mixed, the formulas have a limited lifespan and should be infused according to manufacturers' instructions with any remaining formulas discarded.

Protein

Protein is provided in the form of synthetic amino acids at a standard rate of 1.3–1.5 g/kg ideal body weight/day, a dose that appears to be the minimum required to limit catabolism. A standard solution containing essential and non-essential amino acids is suitable for the vast majority of patients.

Parenteral nutrition should include supplementation of glutamine, a conditionally essential amino acid thought to be involved in a variety of immune processes. A number of trials have demonstrated a reduction in mortality or morbidity with glutamine supplementation doses of 10–30 g/day. Although results are conflicting no trial has shown any suggestion of harm in association with its use. Due to its instability in solution, a dipeptide form of glutamine is used, and if not administered with the PN formula (it is a component of some), may be given separately as an intravenous solution. The addition of glutamine dipeptide may significantly increase daily costs of nutrition support.

Carbohydrate

Although carbohydrate is not considered essential for adequate nutrition, certain tissues, such as brain and red blood cells, are entirely or heavily dependent upon an adequate glucose supply for function. Although this can be supplied by gluconeogenesis from glycogen, fats, and amino acids, this will exacerbate the breakdown of skeletal muscle that already occurs in critical illness. Conventionally, therefore, carbohydrate in the form of glucose is used to provide a large proportion of energy requirements, with a minimum of 2 g/kg/day recommended in current guidelines. In the context of critical illness, insulin resistance impairs glucose uptake and reduces the braking effect of insulin on gluconeogenesis, such that providing even basal glucose requirements may fail to prevent muscle breakdown and hyperglycemia. Exogenous insulin administration is therefore usually required. This may be provided separately or, in a patient with a stable PN and insulin regime, added to custom parenteral formulas.

Lipids

Lipid is indicated as a component of PN firstly to supply calories and secondly to prevent deficiency of the essential fatty acids linoleic acid and alpha-linolenic acid. Lipids generally account for 15–30% of total calorie intake in total parenteral nutrition formulas at a rate of 0.7–1.5 g/kg/day.

Soybean oil was the first source of lipids for PN and it continues to be commonly used. It provides lipid only in the form of long-chain triglycerides. It also provides large amounts of the omega-6 fatty acid linoleic acid, thought to be relatively pro-inflammatory due to its role as a precursor of arachidonic acid. Many commercially available formulations now make use of mixtures of soybean, safflower, coconut, and fish oils with a higher ratio of omega-3 to omega-6 fatty acids and of a mixture of medium-chain and long-chain triglycerides. There is some limited evidence of improvement in markers of inflammation, liver function, immune function, and endothelial function in patients fed with mixtures of medium-chain and long-chain triglycerides, but currently no evidence of clinically significant benefit. The use of fish oil-containing parenteral nutrition in critically ill patients on the other hand, is associated with reduced length of hospital stay as well as improvements in respiratory function and inflammatory burden in numerous studies of critically ill patients, including those with intra-abdominal sepsis and acute pancreatitis, and it is recommended in current ESPEN guidelines.

Micronutrients

Micronutrients (vitamins and trace elements) should be routinely added to parenteral nutrition solutions. Instability in solution may necessitate the addition of a micronutrient solution to commercially available formulas, or the solution may be supplied as a separate pouch in a multi-pouch pack designed for mixing at the bedside. Standard doses of micronutrients are based on the requirements for non-critically ill patients, and the requirements for individual trace elements may be increased in ICU patients, particularly those with high metabolic rate (burns, sepsis) and those receiving renal replacement therapy. Deficiencies are difficult to detect clinically, and monitoring of micronutrient levels is prudent in those with pre-existing malnutrition, with high metabolic demands, receiving renal replacement therapy, and where parenteral nutrition continues for more than 7 days. Given the potential for significant delay in return of these laboratory results, additional supplementation may have to start concurrent with sampling in those most at risk.

Selenium deficiency is common in intensive care, and may be associated with increased tissue susceptibility to oxidative stress. Supplementation of selenium above the level found in standard preparations is indicated in critically ill patients receiving PN for longer than a few days.

Thiamine deficiency is another relatively common problem, particularly in malnourished patients, those with alcohol dependence, and those receiving renal replacement therapy, and may be precipitated by administration of glucose in PN. As well as Wernicke–Korsakoff syndrome, thiamine deficiency is a cause of unexplained lactic acidosis and cardiac failure. In patients at risk, thiamine supplementation should be given prior to the commencement of parenteral nutrition.

Electrolytes

Fluid and electrolyte requirements vary hugely in critically ill patients, and while standard parenteral formulas supply 'typical' requirements for relatively stable patients, frequent monitoring of electrolyte levels is mandatory and daily adjustment of electrolyte content, at least for the first few days, is the rule rather than the exception. That said, PN is not an appropriate route for the primary management of rapidly changing electrolyte levels.

Osmolality

All parenteral formulas are hypertonic and are associated with risk of phlebitis if infused via a peripheral vein. Standard solutions typically have an osmolality greater than 900 mOsm/L, although solutions with an osmolality less than 850 mOsm/L, designed specifically for peripheral use, are available. These solutions are rarely sufficient to meet caloric and nitrogen needs within a reasonable fluid intake volume, and their role in ICU patients is largely confined to supplementation of inadequate enteral nutrition, or as a bridge, either to establishment of central venous access for total parenteral nutrition, or to gut recovery in a malnourished patient. Similarly, their use for more than short periods in ward patients risks volume overload and nutritional deficiency, especially in the elderly or very catabolic patients, and necessitates frequent medical review (Table 6.2).

Selecting the right PN formula for your patient

For the majority of intensive care units, other than those in very small hospitals, custom prescription of TPN is the usual practice. This typically involves admixture of a lipid emulsion, a glucose solution, an amino acid solution, a vitamin and trace element solution, and electrolytes to match each patient's requirement for nutrition, electrolytes, and fluid. A typical formulation might include 25 kCal per kg body weight, with 2 g/kg dextrose, 1.5 g/kg of a standard amino acid solution including 20 g glutamine, and the remainder made up with a lipid emulsion to a total of 1500–2300 mL fluid to be infused over 24 hours. This should also include a standard dose of micronutrients, and sodium, potassium, calcium, and magnesium according to serum levels. When custom PN is unavailable, standard formulations may be considered. A limited range of these is currently available in the United Kingdom and are listed in Table 6.2.

Summary points

- Enteral nutrition should provide 20–30 kCal/kg/day.
- Enteral arginine supplementation may benefit post-operative patients.
- Parenteral nutrition should be commenced if enteral nutrition is contraindicated or energy intake insufficient.
- Parenteral carbohydrates are administered at a rate of 2 g/kg/day, lipids 0.7–1.5 g/kg/day and protein 1.3–1.5 g/kg/day.
- Micronutrients, vitamins, and glutamine should be added to parenteral nutrition.

Table 6.2 Components of selected parenteral nutrition formulations

Convenience products (all quantities per 1000 mL)

Manufacturer	Product name	Energy (KCal)	Carbohydrate (g)	Lipid	Amino acids	Sodium (mmol)	Potassium (mmol)	Osmolality	Trace elements	Vitamins	Glutamine	Arginine (g)
Baxter	Triomel Peripheral	700	75 g glucose (43%)	30 g (43%)	25.3 g (14% total energy)	21	16	760	None	None	None	2.48
Baxter	Triomel 7 g/L with electrolytes, emulsion for infusion	1140	140 g glucose (49% total energy)	40 g olive/soyabean oil (35% total energy)	44.3 g (16% total energy)	35	30	1360	None	None	None	4.34
Baxter	OLICLINOMEL N 5–800 E, emulsion for infusion	915	100 g glucose (44% total energy)	40 g olive/soyabean oil (44% total energy)	28 g (16% total energy)	32	24	995	None	None	None	3.22
Baxter	CLINIMIX® N9G20E, solution for infusion	510	100 g glucose (78% total energy)	None	28 g (22% total energy)	35	30	980	None	None	None	6.32
Fresenius Kabi	Kabiven Peripheral	694	67 g glucose (37% total energy)	35.4 g soybean oil (53% total energy)	23.6 g (10% total energy)	22	17	830	None	None	None	2.36
Fresenius Kabi	Kabiven	877	97 g glucose (42% total energy)	39 g soybean oil (47% total energy)	33 g (11% total energy)	31	24	1230	None	None	None	3.3
Fresenius Kabi	Structokabiven	1066	127 g glucose (45% total energy)	38 g soybean oil (38% total energy)	51 g (17% total energy)	41	30	1610	None	None	None	6.1

Component products: amino acid solutions

Manufacturer	Product name	Contents
Baxter	Synthamin 14, 8.5% intravenous infusion without electrolytes	8.5% amino acid solution. 14 g nitrogen per 1000 mL
Fresenius Kabi	Vamin 14 EF	8.5% amino acid solution. 13.5 g nitrogen per 1000 mL
Fresenius Kabi	Aminoven 25	Concentrated amino acid solution. 25.7 g nitrogen per 1000 mL
Fresenius Kabi	Glamin	Amino acid solution with 20 g/L supplemental glutamine. 18.4 g nitrogen per 1000 mL

Table 6.2 (cont.)

Component products: lipid emulsions

Manufacturer	Product name	Contents
Fresenius Kabi	Intralipid 20%	Soybean oil 200 g/L emulsion. 2000 kcal/L
Fresenius Kabi	SMOFlipid	30% soybean oil, 30% medium-chain triglycerides, 25% olive oil, 15% fish oil. 200 g/L. Energy content 2000 kcal/L
Fresenius Kabi	Structolipid	Mixture of medium and long-chain triglycerides. 200 g/L. Energy content 1960 kcal/L
Baxter	ClinOleic 20% lipid emulsion	Mixture of olive oil (approx 80%) and soyabean oil (approx 20%). Energy content 2000 kcal/L
Fresenius Kabi	Omegaven	10% fish oil emulsion. 10 g/100 mL. Energy content 112 kcal/100 mL

Additives

Manufacturer	Product name	Contents
Fresenius Kabi	Dipeptivan	Glutamine solution, 13.5 g per 100 mL
Fresenius Kabi	Solvito	10 mL vial of water-soluble vitamin mix (B complex vitamins, folic acid, and vitamin C). Equivalent to normal adult daily requirement
Fresenius Kabi	Vitlipid	10 mL vial of fat-soluble vitamin emulsion (vitamins A, D, E, and K). Equivalent to normal adult daily requirement
Fresenius Kabi	Additrace	10 mL vial of trace elements (copper, selenium, manganese, chromium, molybdenum, iron, iodine, fluorine, zinc). Equivalent to normal adult daily requirement

Further reading

Andrews PJD, Avenell A, Noble DW, et al. Randomised trial of glutamine, selenium, or both, to supplement parenteral nutrition for critically ill patients. BMJ 2011;342:d1542.

de Aguilar-Nascimento JE, Prado Silveira BR, Dock-Nascimento DB. Early enteral nutrition with whey protein or casein in elderly patients with acute ischemic stroke: a double-blind randomized trial. Nutrition 2011;27(4):440–444.

Drover JW, Dhaliwal R, Weitzel L, et al. Perioperative use of arginine-supplemented diets: a systematic review of the evidence. J Am Coll Surg 2011;212(3):385–399.e1.

Halmos EP, Muir JG, Barrett JS, et al. Diarrhoea during enteral nutrition is predicted by the poorly absorbed short-chain carbohydrate (FODMAP) content of the formula. Aliment Pharmacol Ther 2010;32(7):925–933.

Heyland DK, Dhaliwal R, Drover JW, et al. Canadian clinical practice guidelines for nutrition support in mechanically ventilated, critically ill adult patients. J Parenter Enteral Nutr 2003:27(5):355–373.

Heyland D, Muscedere J, Wischmeyer PE, et al. A randomized trial of glutamine and antioxidants in critically ill patients. N Engl J Med 2013;368(16):1489–1497.

Kreymann KG, Berger MM, Deutz NEP, et al. ESPEN Guidelines on Enteral Nutrition: intensive care. Clin Nutr 2006;25(2):210–223.

Plauth M, Schütz T. Branched-chain amino acids in liver disease: new aspects of long known phenomena. Curr Opin Clin Nutr Metab Care 2011;14(1):61–66.

Rice TW, Wheeler AP, Thompson BT, et al. Enteral omega-3 fatty acid, gamma-linolenic acid, and antioxidant supplementation in acute lung injury. JAMA 2011;306(14):1574–1581.

Singer P, Berger MM, Van den Berghe G, et al. ESPEN Guidelines on Parenteral Nutrition: intensive care. Clin Nutr 2009;28(4):387–400.

7

Nutritional supplements in critically ill patients

Shaul Lev, Ilya Kagan, and Pierre Singer

Introduction

Evidence has steadily accumulated in favor of the use of nutritional supplements in the support of critically ill patients. The observed effects of nutrients on the immune and inflammatory response have led to the evolution of more sophisticated nutritional concepts and strategies in the critically ill. Acute critical illness is characterized by an accelerated and unbalanced catabolism of proteins, fat, and glycogen stores with the main impediment of physiological function related to protein loss. Protein stores are degraded by the body due to increased energy needs (caloric starvation), new protein needs (amino acids shortage for synthesis of acute phase proteins), hyper-glycosylation, and oxidation. Strategies to reduce protein breakdown include tight caloric supplementation, providing high biological protein supplementation, and avoiding high plasma glucose levels. However, basic nutritional support is only ameliorating, but not stopping the loss of total body protein mass observed in acute severe illness.

Administration of immune-enhancing formulas supplemented with a combination of glutamine, arginine, omega-3 fatty acids, and nucleotides has been shown in many studies to improve infectious outcomes. Reducing inflammation and replenishing the body's antioxidative stores is one of the main goals of nutritional supplementation in critically ill patients. Furthermore, enteral formulas enriched with arginine, nucleotides, glutamine, and omega-3 fatty acids are constantly being investigated in the context of trauma, ARDS, acute pancreatitis, and sepsis. In the present chapter we will focus mainly on substrates designed to diminish oxidative stress and on nutritional supplements aiming towards modulation of the immune system (pharmaco-nutrition).

Immunonutrition

Any nutritional formulation that may modulate the immune response may be referred to as immunonutrition. Pharmaco-nutrition is the science investigating

Nutrition in Critical Care, ed. Peter Faber and Mario Siervo. Published by Cambridge University Press. © Cambridge University Press 2014.

the effects of specific nutrients on the inflammatory and immune responses. Formulations enriched in arginine, omega-3 fatty acids, glutamine, and nucleotides were, and still are, under intensive investigation in different clinical settings related to critical illness.

Omega-3 fatty acids

The omega-3 long-chain fatty acids are a family of biologically active fatty acids. The most biologically active are the very long-chain eicosapentaenoic acid (EPA) and docosahexaenoic acid (DHA). By changing membrane composition these molecules affect membrane fluidity, cell signaling processes, gene expression, and lipid and peptide mediators. EPA and DHA are also substrates for production of biologically potent lipid mediators called resolvins and protectins, which are anti-inflammatory and inflammation resolving. The anti-inflammatory effects of marine n-3 PUFAs suggest that they may be useful as therapeutic agents in disorders with an inflammatory component.

Randomized controlled studies have reported a significant mortality risk reduction, a reduction in the risk of developing new organ failure, and a decrease in time requiring mechanical ventilation for acute lung injury or acute respiratory distress syndrome (ALI/ARDS) patients who received EPA + GLA. Such findings have been confirmed in a meta-analysis demonstrating a significant reduction in the risk of mortality as well as relevant improvements in oxygenation and clinical outcomes of ventilated patients with ALI/ARDS. Recently, however, these results were challenged by the results of the OMEGA study which randomized patients developing acute lung injury to twice daily enteral supplementation of n-3 fatty acids, γ-linolenic acid, and antioxidants compared with an isocaloric-control. The study was stopped early for reasons of futility. An eight-fold increase in plasma eicosapentaenoic acid levels was observed in the study group while the control group received five times more protein intake. Additionally, the use of the n-3 supplement resulted in more patient days with diarrhea. The ESPEN enteral guidelines published in 2006 give grade b recommendation on the use of omega-3 fatty acids in fish oil in patients with ALI/ARDS: "Patients with ARDS should receive EN enriched with n-3 fatty acids and antioxidants (B)".

Fish oil supplementation has been investigated in the setting of acute pancreatitis. Patients that were enrolled to receive parenteral nutrition enriched with 0.15–0.2 g/kg/day fish oil for 5 days had a significantly higher EPA concentration, lower CRP level, and better oxygenation index. Moreover, the number of days of continuous renal replacement therapy in the omega-3 group was significantly less than that in the control group.

These preliminary results suggest that the systemic response to pancreatic and organ injury is attenuated by EPA and DHA. In the meantime, no formal recommendations regarding omega-3 supplementation in acute pancreatitis have been published.

Arginine

L-arginine is an abundant amino acid in body fluids that has a unique role in immune homeostasis. It has been found to be involved in the regulation of T-cells and lymphocytic macrophage cells. Furthermore, arginine deficiency may contribute to microvascular dysfunction and with endothelial nitric oxide being a component in regulating this response. The arginine-to-dimethylarginine ratio is reduced in patients with severe sepsis and is associated with the severity of illness and outcomes. Therefore, it has been suggested that L-arginine supplementation may be of clinical benefit. However, pharmacological manipulation via L-arginine supplementation has so far provided inconsistent clinical results.

Studies of immune-modulating nutrition were mainly carried out in the late 1990s and a meta-analysis published on these trials suggested no effect on mortality in elective surgical patients although the incidence of infections and length of stay were significantly reduced.

In one meta-analysis of critically ill patients, trend was found towards increased mortality especially for patients given formulas that were not enriched with arginine. In this population, a reduced length of stay was also shown with no effect on the rate of infectious complications. Based on these results it was concluded that immune-modulating nutrition could not be recommended generally for the critically ill.

Nucleotides

Nucleotides, which contain a purine or pyridimine base in the nucleic acid structure, serve as building blocks for DNA, RNA, and ATP and are coenzyme components of flavin adenine dinucleotide (FAD), nicotinamide adenine dinucleotide (NAD), and coenzyme-A. Nucleotides are available through de novo synthesis from amino acid precursors or an energy-dependent pathway which involves linkage of a ribose phosphate moiety to available free bases (the rate-limiting factor). Rapidly dividing cells rely heavily on this pathway.

Supplementation of nucleotides enhances lymphocyte blastogenesis, decreases bacterial translocation, and modulates host response against allografts. This has been demonstrated as improved cardiac allograft survival in animals fed a nucleotide-free diet. Nucleotide supplementation may also alter the intestinal microflora environment by acting as a pre-biotic. Reduced infection rates have been reported in infants receiving nucleotide supplemented formulas. Nucleotide supplementation is thought to mitigate the effects of endotoxin-induced intestinal mucosa damage and to reduce bacterial translocation. The clinical data regarding pure enteral nucleotide supplementation is sparse. No randomized prospective studies have been done examining the effect of pure nucleotide supplementation in critically ill patients and thus, no recommendations can be made regarding this specific supplement. One study has reported on a reduction in TPN-induced mucosal atrophy and permeability after supplementation of nucleotides.

Glutamine

Glutamine plays an important role as a carrier for nitrogen and carbon between organs, promotes tissue and cell protection, constitutes part of the anti-oxidant glutathione, and assists in balancing tissue levels of ATP/ADP. Glutamine is also a precursor of several nucleotides, a stimulant for renal angiogenesis, and has been demonstrated to improve intestinal mucosal integrity. In the last two decades, mainly in Europe, therapeutic intravenous glutamine supplementation has been widely used as part of parenteral nutrition in critically ill patients. Although under normal conditions glutamine is described as a non-essential amino acid and its endogenous production is predominantly by skeletal muscle in the range of 50–80 g/24 hours, in situations of severe catabolic state the increase in glutamine demands exceeds endogenous production with a resultant decrease in plasma and tissue glutamine concentrations. Studies have demonstrated that glutamine provides stress tolerance and protection by reducing the release of pro-inflammatory cytokines, specifically interleukin-6 (IL-6) and tumor necrosis factor-α (TNF-α). Recent data show that glutamine activates intracellular signaling pathways and regulates the expression of genes related to signal transduction, apoptosis, and metabolism.

Numerous studies report on the association between glutamine administration, patient reduced mortality and morbidity, decreased time requiring mechanical ventilation, reduction in infections, and improved glucose control. There are no studies showing negative effects of glutamine infusion in critically ill patients and glutamine doses in the range 10–30 g in 24 hours were well tolerated. The route of glutamine administration is still unequivocal. Most studies have investigated parenteral glutamine supplementation. The plasma concentration of glutamine after enteral administration remained low. Recent clinical guidelines of nutrition in critically ill patients recommend intravenous administration of glutamine (Grade A recommendation). ESPEN guidelines recommend glutamine at a dose of 0.2–0.4 g/kg/day for all patients who require parenteral nutrition. In their study, Weitzel and Wischmeyer (2012) recommend larger doses of glutamine (> 0.35–0.5 g/kg/day). Recommendations are based on current meta-analyses that demonstrate a survival benefit in patients receiving these glutamine supplements. Glutamine supplementations can be administered with TPN or safely via a peripheral line.

Selenium (Se), zinc (Zn), and copper (Cu)

The ions and trace elements Se, Zn, Cu, iron, and magnesium (Mg) all play important roles as co-factors required for the antioxidant functions of enzymes like superoxide dismutase, catalase, and glutathione. Glutathione peroxidase is one of the most important enzymes of the antioxidant family. Selenium is an essential trace element of this group of antioxidants and the decrease in plasma glutathione peroxidase activity is correlated with low plasma selenium concentrations. Decreased tissue selenium levels negatively affect cell-mediated and humoral immune function, the activity of natural killer cells, and the ability of free radical neutralization. Selenium availability and requirements are affected by several factors, e.g., the nutritional environment, statins, glucocorticoids, smoking, alcoholism, and AIDS may all be associated with reductions in blood and tissue selenium levels. Also, independently, due to the capillary leakage and redistribution of trace elements from the circulation to the interstitial space in SIRS, selenium plasma concentration decreases markedly. Other factors that influence selenium levels in critically ill patients are the depletions of selenium observed through extensive losses from, e.g., burns, diarrhea, fistulae, vomiting, polyuria, drains, open abdominal losses, renal replacement therapy, and importantly an inadequate supply of selenium in enteral or parenteral nutrition. Several trials have shown beneficial effects such as a decrease in complications from infection and organ dysfunction and reduced in-hospital mortality in patients receiving selenium supplementation. However, optimal safe doses and route of administration remain controversial. Doses of selenium between 1000 µg/day and 1600 µg/day have all reported beneficial effects.

Zinc is an essential trace element contributing to immune response, metabolic processes such as glucose control, glutathione activity, and wound healing. It follows that low plasma and tissue concentrations of zinc have been linked to immune dysfunction, increased infection rates, and increased morbidity and mortality in critically ill patients, especially the subgroup of septic patients. The decrease in zinc plasma concentration can partially be explained by the redistribution of carrier proteins (especially albumin) due to changes in vascular permeability, loss from surgical drains, urine, and sequestration into tissues and mucosal secretions. As no studies have clearly demonstrated a significant change in mortality or length of stay in patients receiving zinc supplementation, there is currently no data on an optimal dose of zinc to be included in antioxidant supplementation.

Despite the firm lack of evidence zinc and selenium are both recommended as trace elements in formulas together with copper, magnesium, and other micronutrients. Recent European and American nutrition guidelines for critically ill patients recommend a daily dose of trace elements and multivitamins. The doses of microelements should be adapted in proportion to the other nutritional requirements and relate to the underlying symptoms and disease. In special situations, for example in chronically critically ill patients or in patients undergoing continuous renal replacement therapy, determination of plasma level may be considered for detection of deficiencies and individual corrections of trace elements may be required.

Trace element dosages in standard formulations are very variable with multifold variations, e.g., selenium ranges between 20 and 70 µg/mL and zinc between 3.7 and 10 mg/mL. The ESPEN guidelines on parenteral nutrition recommend that the selenium dose in critically ill patients should not exceed 750–1000 µg/day. Recommendations from ASPEN are 100–400 µg/day of selenium in the critically ill patient. However, this might require adjustment in, for example, patients with major burns (> 20% of body surface) who suffer from large exudative losses of copper, selenium, and zinc, as randomized trials demonstrate benefits from doses calculated to compensate for these losses (3–3.5 mg Cu, 30–35 mg Zn, and 350 µg Se per day for 2–3 weeks). Furthermore, in patients receiving continuous renal replacement therapy additional doses of selenium and zinc should be administered.

Summary points

- In selected groups of patients omega-3 fatty acid supplementation may reduce the risk of infection and time of mechanical ventilation.
- L-Arginine supplementation has not provided any significant clinical benefits in critically ill patients.
- Glutamine is a ubiquitous amino acid involved in immune function and anti-oxidant defenses. Glutamine supplementation results in a reduction in morbidity and mortality.
- There are clinical benefits to supplementation of trace elements. Dosage might require adjustment in selected patient groups.

Further reading

Duncan A, Dean P, Simm M, O'Reilly DS, Kinsella J. Zinc supplementation in intensive care: results of a UK survey. J Crit Care 2012;27:102.e1–102.e6.

Hardy G, Hardy I, Manzanares W. Selenium supplementation in the critically ill. Nutr Clin Pract 2012;27:21–33.

Heyland D, Novak F, Drover JW, Jain M, Su X, Suchner U. Should immunonutrition become routine in critically ill patients? JAMA 2001;286:944–953.

Kreymann KG, Berger MM, Deutz NE, et al. ESPEN guidelines on enteral nutrition: intensive care. Clin Nutr 2006;25:210–223.

Pontes-Arruda A, Demichele S, Seth A, Singer P. The use of an inflammation-modulating diet in patients with acute lung injury or acute respiratory distress syndrome: a meta-analysis of outcome data. J Parenter Enteral Nutr 2006;32:596–605.

Reddel L, Cotton BA. Antioxidants and micronutrient supplementation in trauma patients. Curr Opin Clin Nutr Metab Care 2012;15:181–187.

Rice TW, Wheeler AP, Thompson BT, et al. Enteral omega-3 fatty acid, gamma-linolenic acid, and antioxidant supplementation in acute lung injury. JAMA 2011;306:1574–1581.

Santora R, Kozar RA. Molecular mechanism of pharmaconutrients. J Surg Res 2010;161:288–294.

Singer P, Berger MM, van den Berghe G, et al. ESPEN Guidelines on Parenteral Nutrition: intensive care. Clin Nutr 2009;28:327–400.

Wang X, Li W, Zhang F, Pan L, Li N, Li J. Fish oil-supplemented parenteral nutrition in severe acute pancreatitis patients and effects on immune function and infectious risk: a randomized controlled trial. Inflammation 2009;32:304–309.

Weitzel LR, Wischmeyer PE. Glutamine in critical illness: The time has come, the time is now. Crit Care Clin 2012;26:515–525.

Wernerman J. Glutamine supplementation. Ann Intensive Care 2011;12(1):25.

General Problems in Critical Care

8

Gastrointestinal disturbances in critically ill patients

Andrew M. Hetreed and Peter Faber

Introduction

Assessment of mechanical and physiological GI function in critically ill patients is at most times difficult and in practical terms limited to clinical signs, examination, and what are effectively enhanced input-output measurements from which to draw conclusions. The compound impression from clinical observations and laboratory tests is usually sufficient to consider the functional integrity of the GI tract and how well or badly it is performing in the individual patient. There is evidence that the presence of GI symptoms in critically ill patients affects outcome but it is notable that in the few studies which have been performed there is significant variability in the reported incidence of symptoms. This is at least in part due to a lack of universally agreed definitions as to what constitutes a significant GI symptom, and variations in the assessment of failing GI function. The lack of any objective tests which can be performed to evaluate performance and functional reserve of the GI tract compounds this problem. Studies have reported that approximately 60% of intensive care patients will have at least one GI symptom during their stay and amongst those with multiple symptoms, GI bleeding or absent bowel sounds is associated with increased morbidity and mortality.

The European Society of Intensive Care Medicine (ESICM) Working Group on Abdominal Problems has published recommendations on terminology, definitions, and management of GI disturbances in the critically ill population. These definitions and terminology are used in the following discussions on gastrointestinal problems of critical care patients.

Acute gastrointestinal injury

Acute gastrointestinal injury (AGI) is malfunctioning of the GI tract in critically ill patients due to their acute illness, and is graded according

Nutrition in Critical Care, ed. Peter Faber and Mario Siervo. Published by Cambridge University Press. © Cambridge University Press 2014.

Table 8.1 Gastrointestinal dysfunction.

	Definition	Example
Grade I (risk of developing gastrointestinal dysfunction or failure)	The function of the GI tract is partially impaired, expressed as GI symptoms related to a known cause and perceived as transient	Nausea/vomiting in the immediate post-operative period, absent bowel sounds after abdominal surgery
Grade II (gastrointestinal dysfunction)	The GI tract is not able to perform digestion and absorption adequately to satisfy the nutrient and fluid requirements of the body. There are no changes in general condition of the patient related to GI problems	Gastroparesis with high gastric residuals, diarrhea, grade 1 intra-abdominal hypertension (IAP 12–15 mmHg), visible blood in gastric content or stool, feeding intolerance*
Grade III (gastrointestinal failure)	Loss of GI function, where restoration of GI function is not achieved despite interventions and the general condition is not improving	Persistent feeding intolerance, GI paralysis, bowel dilatation, grade 2 IAH (IAP 16–20 mmHg), bowel ischemia
Grade IV (gastrointestinal failure with severe impact on distant organ function)	AGI has progressed to become directly and immediately life threatening, with worsening of MODS and shock	Bowel necrosis, abdominal compartment syndrome (IAP > 20 mmHg), hemorrhagic shock from GI bleeding

*Feeding intolerance is present if at least 20 kcal/kg/day cannot be given via enteral route within 72 hours of attempted feeding.
MODS, multi-organ dysfunction score.

to severity in a manner similar to the grading of acute kidney injury (Table 8.1).

In addition, AGI may be further defined as primary or secondary: primary AGI is associated with primary disease or direct injury to organs of the GI system, while secondary AGI develops as a consequence of a host response in critical illness without primary pathology of the GI system.

Diarrhea

The passing of three or more loose or liquid stools (Bristol Stool Chart 5, 6, or 7) with total mass greater than 250 g or total volume greater than 250 mL per day constitutes diarrhea. The reported incidence of diarrhea on critical care units varies from 2–95% and has proven difficult to establish with certainty. A 2011 multi-center Spanish study reported a mean prevalence of 6.4% amongst critical care patients.

Risk factors for diarrhea

- Enteral nutrition (odds ratio 4.1)
- Antibiotic therapy
- Increasing ICU length of stay
- Hyperglycemia
- Hypoalbuminemia
- Elevated WCC
- *Clostridium difficile* infection

Management

The mainstay of therapy is symptomatic management, with maintenance of appropriate fluid status and electrolyte balance to prevent secondary deterioration (e.g., renal dysfunction). A fecal collection system (e.g., Flexiseal™) reduces the risk of peri-anal skin damage and bed sores, and can be used if the stool is type 7. The addition of soluble fiber to enteral feeding solutions prolongs transit time and may alleviate symptoms.

A cause should be sought and treated if possible (e.g., pro-kinetics, antibiotics, inflammatory bowel disease, malabsorption). The routine sending of stool cultures is rarely of value for patients admitted to the intensive care unit. Instead stool should be sent for analysis of *C. difficile* endotoxin and culture for pathogens considered if results are negative and diarrhea persistent. Routine stool culture will identify *Salmonella*, *Campylobacter*, and *Shigella* species. If there is clinical suspicion of other pathogens the laboratory should be notified and local guidelines implemented. The examination of stool samples for ova and parasites (e.g., for *Giardia*, *Cryptosporidium*, *Cyclospora*, and *Entamoeba hystolytica*) may be appropriate if the patient has a history of foreign travel or immuno-suppression. Testing for these is done by collecting three samples sent for analysis at least 24 hours apart since parasite excretion may be intermittent.

Where *C. difficile* is isolated, metronidazole is as effective as oral vancomycin unless the infection is recurrent or severe. Specific dosing will depend on local policies, but 10–14 days of therapy with oral/nasogastric (NG) metronidazole 400 mg three times a day is often sufficient, and if treatment fails 10–14 days of oral/NG vancomycin 125–250 mg four times a day can be considered.

Vomiting (emesis)

Any visible regurgitation of gastric contents, regardless of the amount, constitutes vomiting. The common definition of vomiting outside the critical care unit requires contractions of the gut and abdominal wall musculature to produce oral expulsion of

GI contents; however in ICU patients, these involuntary, muscular contractions are often not detectable. Therefore, in the ICU population vomiting and regurgitation should be considered together. In the absence of physical obstruction, impaired gastric emptying is the likely etiology and is considered in the next section.

In contrast to conscious patients outside the critical care environment the sensation of nausea is less of an issue than any regurgitation that may occur, as patients are often sedated or anesthetized within the ICU. Hence, the role of commonly used anti-emetics such as cyclizine or 5-HT$_3$ antagonists (ondansetron, granisetron etc.) is reduced, and they are only likely to be of value in conscious patients or where forceful emesis is occurring.

Hypomotility

The proportion of ventilated patients exhibiting antral hypomotility, reduced gastric emptying, and diminished migrating motor complexes is approaching 50%, leading to a multitude of problems – not least of which is the reduced ability to tolerate enteral nutrition. Hypomotility can usefully be divided into gastroparesis and intestinal motor inhibition; though obviously these can, and often do, coexist in the same patient.

Gastroparesis

Gastroparesis is impaired gastric emptying without physical obstruction, and can be assessed by the quantity of gastric aspirate obtained over a set period. Gastric juice can be assumed to be produced at a rate of approximately 1 L/day, and the amount of it passing through the pyloric sphincter can therefore be estimated as the volume which is not aspirated.

Intestinal motor inhibition

Intestinal motor inhibition refers to disruption of the basic patterns of propulsion seen in the small and large bowel. These are controlled primarily by integrated reflex circuits in the enteric nervous system, the activity of the interstitial cells of Cajal (the 'pacemakers' of the bowel), and the smooth muscle cells themselves. Modulation of motility by the autonomic nervous system and endocrine messengers provides fine tuning of propulsive activity. In critical illness any or all of these systems can become disrupted, and restoration of normal function can be very difficult.

Outside the critical care environment constipation implies uncomfortable or infrequent bowel movements with hard stool and/or painful defecation. Because these symptoms may not be expressed in critical care patients the term "paralysis of the lower gastrointestinal tract" has been suggested. This is the inability of the bowel to pass stool due to impaired peristalsis.

Clinical signs include absence of stool for three or more consecutive days without mechanical obstruction, though it is worth remembering that physiological stool frequency can vary from one to two evacuations per day to one evacuation every third or fourth day. Bowel sounds may or may not be present.

Management of hypomotility

Management can be divided into initial supportive therapeutic options and goal-directed specific therapies. A cohesive standardized approach was proposed by Herbert & Holzer in 2008 and forms the basis for these recommendations.

Conditions impairing peristalsis (e.g., hypokalemia, hyperglycemia) should be corrected and drugs reducing GI motility (e.g., opioids, sedatives, catecholamines) stopped wherever possible. To be of use laxative drugs must be either given prophylactically or started early owing to their delayed onset of action. Tables 8.2 and Table 8.3 illustrate guidance on stimulant and osmotic laxatives.

Supportive therapy

Bisacodyl must be activated by hydrolysis by endogenous esterases in the bowel resulting in a 6–12 hour delay until the effects of an oral dose are observed. In contrast, administration as a suppository can produce laxation within 60 minutes and avoids enterohepatic circulation. Picosulfate is hydrolyzed to its active form by colonic bacteria.

Macrogol 3350 is dissolved in an electrolyte-balanced solution, creating a watery bulk which distends the bowel wall and is likely to trigger peristalsis. Lactulose should be used with caution – it is a synthetic disaccharide which passes unchanged through the small bowel and is fermented in the colon. This can cause massive fluid and fat loss and extensive bloating, which may increase intra-abdominal pressure.

Goal-directed therapies

Erythromycin is a macrolide antibiotic with direct action at motilin receptors on enteric neurons and smooth muscle cells. It is effective in improving gastric emptying, but appears not to reduce colonic transit time and confers no effect in

Table 8.2 Stimulant laxatives

1st line	Bisacodyl	10–20 mg PR
2nd line	Bisacodyl	10–20 mg PO
	Sodium picosulfate	10–20 mg PO

Table 8.3 Osmotic laxatives

1st line	Polyethylene glycol (Macrogol 3350)	20–30 g/day PO
2nd line	Magnesium salts	0.1 mg/kg PO

Table 8.4 Prokinetic medication for gastroparesis

1st line	Erythromycin	100 mg i.v. TDS (3 days maximum)
2nd line	Metoclopramide	10 mg i.v. TDS
3rd line	Domperidone	30–40 mg PO

Table 8.5 Gastroparesis with intestinal motor inhibition

1st line	Erythromycin	100 mg i.v. TDS
	24 h after first dose	(3 days maximum)
	Metoclopramide	10–30 mg IV
	+ Neostigmine	0.5–1.5 mg i.v. OD over 2 h

post-operative ileus. Metoclopramide is a D_2 receptor antagonist, a partial 5-HT_4 receptor agonist, and a weak central and peripheral 5-HT_3 antagonist. 5-HT_4 activation promotes acetylcholine release from enteric neurons and is the likely primary source of metoclopramide's prokinetic activity. It is, however, also ineffective in the treatment of post-operative ileus. Domperidone mediates prokinesis via peripheral dopamine receptor antagonism, and is also a potent anti-emetic. It does not readily cross the blood-brain barrier and therefore does not exhibit the extra-pyramidal side effects sometimes seen with metoclopramide. Tables 8.4 and 8.5 contain dosage guidance for commonly available prokinetics.

Neostigmine is an acetylcholinesterase inhibitor, and its combination with metoclopramide produces greater increase in ACh concentrations within the enteric nervous system than that provided by either alone. Bradycardia may be a problematic side effect and can be treated with vagolytics such as atropine or glycopyrollate. Neostigmine has been used with some success in the treatment of acute colonic pseudo-obstruction (Ogilvie's syndrome), and in this context 2–2.5 mg can be given as an intravenous bolus over 2–3 minutes. A combination preparation with 500 μg glycopyrollate is available.

Peripherally acting mu-opioid receptor antagonists have been used with some success to treat opioid-induced bowel dysfunction with an incidence of adverse events similar to placebo; however, the long-term safety and efficacy of these drugs is yet to be established and currently their routine use is not recommended.

Gastrointestinal bleeding

Blood loss into the lumen of the gastrointestinal tract may be confirmed by the macroscopic presence of blood as hematemesis or melena.

The majority of ICU patients suffer asymptomatic but endoscopically evident damage to GI tract mucosa during their stay with a smaller number, 5–25%, with clinically evident bleeding from the GI tract. Clinically important bleeding, defined as overt bleeding requiring blood transfusion or causing hemodynamic instability, occurs in 1.5–4% of ventilated patients.

Stress ulceration of the upper GI tract begins within hours of the onset of critical illness. Most overt GI bleeding is caused by either gastric or esophageal ulceration.

Management of gastrointestinal bleeding

The management of GI bleeding is determined initially by the hemodynamic status of the patient. If the patient is unstable, urgent endoscopy should be performed and bleeding points stopped either by injection of adrenaline, clipping, banding, or injection of sclerosant. If bleeding cannot be endoscopically controlled interventional radiology should be considered and in rare cases a laparotomy may be required.

A Sengstaken-Blakemore tube is of value for the control of refractory bleeding from esophageal varices – it is important to note that the mechanism of action of this tube is via traction (of approximately 10N) to compress the gastro-esophageal junction and reduce blood flow to the varices. The esophageal balloon is of secondary importance and may be inflated if traction has failed to stop the bleeding. It should not remain inflated for more than 6 hours due to the risk of esophageal ischemia and necrosis.

If the patient is hemodynamically stable endoscopy remains the most appropriate management, albeit with reduced urgency.

The use of pharmacological agents to increase gastric pH in patients with bleeding from gastric ulcers has been examined in several studies, looking at administration both before and after endoscopy. H2-receptor blockers have not been shown to significantly accelerate hemostasis or reduce the rate of bleeding recurrence and are of little value in this context. Proton pump inhibitors are far more effective inhibitors of acid production, and consensus guidelines continue to support the use of high-dose intravenous PPI (80 mg omeprazole bolus followed by 8 mg/hour infusion for 72 hours) in patients with bleeding ulcers, visible vessels, or adherent clot at endoscopy. Alternative high-dose omeprazole, e.g., 40 mg omeprazole i.v. twice daily has been shown to be equivalent in terms of reductions in rebleeding, mortality, and the need for surgery. Commencement of acid suppression prior to endoscopy is associated with identification of fewer actively bleeding ulcers and a reduced need for therapy but does not alter rates of rebleeding or surgery, and may be considered depending on local gastroenterology policy. During the active management of gastrointestinal bleeding any nasogastric feeding would obviously have to be paused but should be re-commenced as soon as clinically indicated.

Abdominal hypertension and compartment syndrome

Definition:
1. Intra-abdominal hypertension (IAH) is present if the intra-abdominal pressure (IAP) is found to be 12 mmHg or more in at least two separate measurements

1–6 hours apart, or if the mean of IAP measurements over 24 hours is 12 mmHg or more (provided at least four measurements were made).
2. Abdominal compartment syndrome (ACS) is defined as a sustained increase in IAP to 20 mmHg or greater, again in at least two separate measurements 1–6 hours apart, with new onset organ failure.

Management of abdominal hypertension

If IAH/ACS is suspected intermittent monitoring of IAP should be under-taken. This is most easily accomplished by transducing the pressure in the urinary bladder after instilling 50 mL of sterile 0.9% saline above a clamped catheter.

In patients with ascites and IAH percutaneous decompression is recommended. Thoracic epidural infusion of local anesthetic may decrease IAP in post-operative patients, and nasogastric/colonic decompression has been suggested for removal of intraluminal contents. Neuromuscular blockade reduces IAP, but may increase patients' risk of aspiration and ventilator-associated pneumonia.

Surgical decompression remains the only definitive management for ACS, though the timeline for surgery has not been well established. It is currently recommended as a life-saving procedure for patients for whom other approaches to reducing IAP have failed, and should be considered prophylactically in patients undergoing high-risk laparotomy (e.g., repair of ruptured AAA (abdominal aortic aneurysm)). Patients with IAH and compartment syndrome will require parenteral nutrition until recovered. Fluid administration should be carefully monitored in these patients to avoid further gastrointestinal and pulmonary edema.

Summary points

- Acute gastrointestinal injury may be primary or secondary, and is graded I–IV according to severity.
- Diarrhea is a common and sometimes unavoidable complication of critical care; management aims to identify a cause and minimize secondary physiological impact.
- The etiology of hypomotility is complex and multifactorial, and as a result treatment can be difficult. Distinction of upper and lower GI paralysis allows more targeted therapies while a multimodal approach including prokinesis and laxation where appropriate is usually most effective.
- GI ulceration is common in critical illness, and may lead to significant GI bleeding. Endoscopic management is the gold standard. The role of acid suppression and its timing with respect to endoscopy is contentious.
- Measurement of IAP should be performed wherever there is suspicion of IAH or abdominal compartment syndrome – if basic therapies fail, definitive management is surgical.

Further reading

Andriulli A, Loperfido S, Focareta R, et al. High- versus low-dose proton pump inhibitors after endoscopic hemostasis in patients with peptic ulcer bleeding: a multicentre, randomized study. Am J Gastroenterol 2008;103(12):3011.

Barkun A, Bardou M, Kuipers E, et al. International consensus recommendations on the management of patients with nonvariceal upper gastrointestinal bleeding. Ann Intern Med 2010;151:101–113.

Cook D, Fuller H, Gyatt G, et al. Risk factors for gastrointestinal bleeding in critically ill patients. N Engl J Med 1994;330:377–381.

Herbert M, Holzer P. Standardized concept for the treatment of gastrointestinal dysmotility in critically ill patients: current status and future options. Clin Nutr 2008;27:25–41.

Jack L, Coyer F, Courtney M, Venkatesh B. Diarrhoea, enteral nutrition and intestinal flora relationships in critically ill patients. Intensive Care Med 2010;36:S330.

Malbrain M, De laet I, Cheatham M. Consensus conference definitions and recommendations on intra-abdominal hypertension and the abdominal compartment syndrome – the long road to the final publications, and how did we get there? Acta Clin Belg Suppl 2007;62:44–59.

McNicol E, Boyce D, Schumann R, Carr D. Efficacy and safety of mu-opioid antagonists in the treatment of opioid-induced bowel dysfunction: systematic review and meta-analysis of randomized controlled trials. Pain Med 2008;9(6):634–659.

Reintam Blaser A, Malbrain M, Starkopf J, et al. Gastrointestinal function in intensive care patients: terminology, definitions and management. Recommendations of the ESICM Working Group on Abdominal Problems. Intensive Care Med 2012;38(3):384–394.

Ritz M, Fraser R, Tam W, Dent J. Impacts and patterns of disturbed gastrointestinal function in critically ill patients. Am J Gastroenterol 2000;95:3044–3052.

Fluid and electrolyte management in critical care medicine

Nils Siegenthaler, Paolo Merlani, and Andreas Perren

Introduction

In critically ill patients fluid and electrolyte management may be complex due to alterations in absorption, excretion and distribution, as well as perturbation of hormonal state and homeostatic process by the pathology or by the treatment needed. Fluid and electrolyte management deals with two interrelated issues: body fluid composition (water and electrolytes) and the hemodynamically effective blood volume.

Clinically applied physiology of fluid and electrolytes in critically ill patients

Total body water (TBW) ranges from 50% to 80% of the lean body mass (BM), depending on age and gender of the patient (Table 9.1). Lean BM must be used for the estimation of TBW since adipose tissue has a low content in water. TBW is distributed in the following spaces: intracellular ($\approx$40% of BM; 28 L for a 70 kg adult), extracellular extravascular or interstitial ($\approx$15%; 10.5 L), and extracellular intravascular ($\approx$5%; 3.5 L). The so-called "third space" (e.g., peritoneal [ascites], pleural) belongs to the interstitial compartment.

The partition between the intracellular and extracellular compartments depends on the osmotic gradient, and the distribution between the intravascular and the interstitial compartment is mainly determined by the Starling's forces:

$$\text{Net filtration of fluid} = L_p \times [(P_{cap} - P_{if}) - s(\Pi_{cap} - \Pi_{if})]$$

Where L_p is the unit of capillary wall permeability, P the hydrostatic pressure of capillaries (cap) and interstitium (if), Π the capillary and interstitial oncotic pressure, and s the coefficient of reflection of protein across the capillary wall.

Nutrition in Critical Care, ed. Peter Faber and Mario Siervo. Published by Cambridge University Press. © Cambridge University Press 2014.

Table 9.1 Amount of total body water according to gender and body mass index

Body mass index	Total body water (% body weight)			
	Infant	Adult (male)	Adult (female)	Elderly
< 22	80	65	60	55
22–30	70	60	55	50
> 30	65	55	50	50

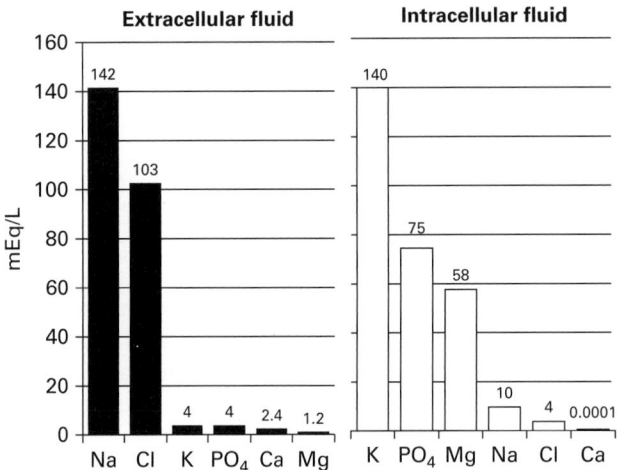

Figure 9.1 Imbalance of osmolality (induced by solutes other than Na) between intracellular and extracellular compartment resulting in a free water shift.

Osmotic pressure (albumin) and vascular permeability are the main determinants of this trans-membrane fluid movement. Clinically relevant electrolytes are mainly sodium (Na), potassium (K), calcium (Ca), magnesium (Mg), and phosphorus (PO$_4$). The partition of electrolytes and body fluid composition in each compartment is summarized in Figure 9.1.

Body fluid and electrolyte homeostasis

To maintain homeostasis, daily loss of water and electrolytes must be replaced with solutions (Table 9.2) of similar composition to the lost fluid (Table 9.3) and this replacement must be assessed with regular laboratory controls.

Daily fluid loss (insensible, gastrointestinal, and renal [0.3 mL/kg/hour]) represents an hourly need of about 60 mL + 1 mL/kg/hour (1700 mL/day for an average adult of 70 kg). In addition, electrolytes lost must be replaced (Na 1–2 mEq/kg/day and K 1–1.5 mEq/kg/day). In order to correct altered body fluid composition,

Table 9.2 Compositions of parenteral and enteral fluid therapy

Solution*	Na (mEq/L)	K (mEq/L)	Osmolality (mmol/kg)
Parenteral solutions			
NaCl 0.45%	77	0	154
NaCl 0.9%	154	0	308
NaCl 3%	513	0	1026
Lactated Ringer	130	4	274
Sodium bicarbonate 8.4%	1000	0	2000
Albumin 5%	150	<2	309
Tetrastarch 6% 130/0.4 (Voluven®)	154	0	308
Parenteral nutrition examples			
Nutriflex® lipid special	52	38	1545
Enteral solutions			
Free water	0	0	NA
Novasource® forte	37	35	328
Promote® fibers	57	51	292

*List is not exhaustive.

Table 9.3 Composition of body fluids

Fluid	Na (mEq/L)	K (mEq/L)	Cl (mEq/L)
Gastric	≈ 60	≈ 10	≈ 130
Duodenum	≈ 140	≈ 5	≈ 80
Bile	≈ 145	≈ 5	≈ 100
Pancreas	≈ 140	≈ 5	≈ 75
Ileum	≈ 140	≈ 5	≈ 104
Colon	≈ 60	≈ 30	≈ 40
Sweat	≈ 40	≈ 5	≈ 40

clinically relevant mechanisms of fluid and electrolyte dysregulation will be discussed (Table 9.4).

Regulation of Na and free water

Na is the main determinant of serum osmolality (Serum osm).

$$\text{Serum osm } (\text{mOsm/Kg H}_2\text{O}) \approx 2[\text{Na:meq/L}] + \text{Glucose[mmol/L]} + \text{BUN[mmol/L]}$$

Thus, perturbation of Na concentration (true hyper- or hyponatremia) is generally associated with similar changes in serum osmolality. Water diffuses freely across compartments according to their respective osmolality and perturbations of serum Na concentration may suggest alterations in both Na and/or water balance or partition between compartments. Remember that every change in Na serum

Table 9.4 Common causes of alteration in body fluid composition

Hypernatremia	A. Na infusion
	● Sodium bicarbonate
	● Hypertonic saline
	B. Water loss
	● Burns, fever, osmotic diarrhea, osmotic diuresis, post-obstructive diuresis
	C. Decreased renal capacity of urine concentration
	● Central diabetes insipidus:
	● Intracerebral lesions, infections
	● Nephrogenic diabetes insipidus:
	● Osmotic diuresis, hypercalcemia, hypokalemia, sickle cell disease, drug treatment (lithium intoxication, amphotericin B)
	D. Other
	● Hyperaldosteronism
Hyponatremia	A. Increase in serum osmolality (hyperosmotic hyponatremia)
	B. Decreased renal perfusion or glomerular filtration rate
	● Intravascular hypovolemia:
	● Absolute hypovolemia (heart failure, bleeding, diarrhea)
	● Relative hypovolemia (cirrhosis, vasoplegia)
	● Renal failure
	B. Decreased NaCl reabsorption
	● Diuretic (thiazides > loop diuretics)
	C. Excess ADH
	● SIADH (meningitis, encephalitis, cerebrovascular accident, head trauma, severe pneumonia, Guillian-Barré syndrome, physical or emotional stress, pain)
	D. Other
	● Adrenal insufficiency
	● Hypothyroidism
Hyperkalemia	A. Excessive K intake
	B. Transcellular shift
	● Metabolic acidemia (mainly other than organic acidosis)
	● Insulin deficiency
	● Digoxin
	● Succinylcholine
	● Hemolysis, rhabdomyolysis
	C. Decreased renal excretion of K
	● Renal failure
	● Hypoaldosteronism or resistance
	● Adrenal insufficiency, ACE inhibitors, NSAIDs, heparin
	● Decreased urine flow in distal nephron

Table 9.4 (cont.)

Hypokalemia	A. Transcellular shift of K
	• Metabolic alkalosis
	• Insulin
	• Beta-agonists (stress, delirium tremens, salbutamol)
	B. Increased renal excretion of K
	• Mineralocorticoid
	• Increased urine flow in the distal nephron
	• Diuretics, osmotic diuresis
	• Non-reabsorbed anion
	• Vomiting, ketoacidosis
	C. Hypomagnesemia
Hypophosphatemia	A. Decreased adsorption
	• Vitamin D deficiency
	B. Transcellular shift
	• Refeeding syndrome, insulin
	C. Renal loss
	• Hyperparathyroidism, osmotic diuresis, continuous hemofiltration
Hyperphosphatemia	A. Transcellular shift
	• Tumor lysis syndrome, hemolysis, rhabdomyolysis
	B. Decreased renal excretion
	• Renal failure, hypoparathyroidism
Hypocalcemia	A. Rhabdomyolysis
	B. Pancreatitis
	C. Hyperphosphatemia
	D. Polytransfusion
Hypercalcemia	A. Malignant (multiple myeloma, lymphoma, lung cancer, breast)
	B. Hyperparathyroidism (primary/tertiary)
	C. Drugs
	• Thiazides, theophylline, lithium
	D. Sarcoidosis/tuberculosis
	E. Immobilization
	F. Hypervitaminosis D and A
	G. Hyperthyroidism
	H. Milk alkali syndrome
Hypomagnesemia	A. Low intakes
	B. Excessive loss
	• Renal: tubular dysfunction, hypercalcemia, osmotic diuresis, diuretics
	• Gastrointestinal: emesis, nasogastric suction, diarrhea
	C. Others
	• Drugs (aminoglycosides, ciclosporin, amphotericin B, cis-platinum)
	• Decompensated diabetes mellitus
	• Refeeding syndromes/parenteral nutrition
Hypermagnesemia	A. Excessive intake /administration
	• In relation to renal insufficiency
	• Therapeutic (pre-/eclampsia)

concentration will be associated with changes in water distribution between intracellular and extracellular compartments: hypernatremia leads to a decrease in cellular fluid volume and hyponatremia to an increase in cellular fluid volume (edema). In the critical care setting, modifications in Na concentration are frequently related to inappropriate infusion or compensation of free water or Na loss with altered renal capacity of urine concentration/dilution.

Inappropriate compensation or infusion of free water and/or Na

When large amounts of free water are lost and not appropriately compensated, hypernatremia may result. Conversely, excessive serum dilution and hyponatremia can be encountered after adsorption of isosmotic solutions containing low Na (during transurethral resection of the prostate). Compensation of free water or Na loss (according to the composition of the fluid lost – Table 9.2), in addition to the estimation of the effect from all kind of infused fluids (e.g., antibiotic containing Na, sodium bicarbonate) are essential to avoid changes in body fluid composition.

Imbalance of osmolality (included by solutes other than Na) between intracellular and extracellular compartment resulting in a free water shift

Hyperosmolality induced by hyperglycemia induces a shift of free water from the intracellular compartment to the extracellular space, resulting in dilutional hyponatremia. This situation represents an exception, as hyponatremia is associated with hyperosmolality. In order to avoid the development of hypernatremia after the correction of hyperglycemia (infusion of Na-containing solution with water shift into the cells) clinicians should predict the Na serum concentration following the correction of hyperglycemia:

$$\text{Corrected Na} = \text{measured Na concentration (mmol/L)} + [\text{serum glucose concentration (mmol/L)} - 5]/3.5$$

During treatment of hyperosmolal (hypernatremia, hyperglycemia) or hypoosmolal states (hyponatremia) an effect of serum osmolality on body fluid repartition needs to be considered. Rapid changes in serum osmolality will result in an increase in intracellular fluid content (cerebral edema) when serum osmolality is decreased too quickly (> 0.5 meq/L/hour) or in intracellular dehydration (possible association with central pontine myelinolysis) when increased too quickly.

Finally, the action of serum osmolality on body fluid repartition may be used in the treatment of critically ill patients. During cerebral edema, intracranial pressure may be lowered by rising serum osmolality with hyperosmotic solution (hypertonic saline or mannitol).

Renal capacity of urine concentration/dilution

In response to changes in Na concentration, the kidneys increase the excretion of water and decrease Na excretion during hyponatremia (urine dilution: urine osmolality < 100–300 mOsm/kg) or vice versa during hypernatremia (urine concentration: urine osmolality > 300–800 mOsml/kg). Perturbation of renal concentration/dilution capacity may result from:

- Decrease in renal perfusion reducing the quantity of free water and Na available for filtration and excretion – During hypovolemia, heart failure, or cirrhosis, where low intravascular volume and/or inadequate distribution of blood flow result in a decreased renal perfusion, free water excretion is impaired and, due to increased anti-diuretic hormone (ADH) release, most of the filtered water is reabsorbed. This may result in hyponatremia if hypotonic solution is infused/ingested.
- Renal failure – Free water or Na must be filtered as urine for being excreted. When renal function is severely decreased, unbalanced load in free water or Na may not be equilibrated, resulting in hypo- or hypernatremia, respectively.
- Capacity of proximal reabsorption of Na – This regulation, partly mediated by aldosterone, allows the generation of dilute urine. Loop diuretics (furosemide) act on the Na-K-2CL carrier in the thick ascending limb. They induce an increase in excretion of Na (and calcium). In contrast to thiazides, loop diuretics decrease the medullary osmolal gradient resulting in a reduced ability of ADH to increase the reabsorption of water and thus limiting the development of hyponatremia. Thiazides act mainly in the distal tubule where Na reabsorption is weak and have a smaller effect on medullary osmolal gradient, resulting in a limited diuretic effect, more frequently associated with hyponatremia. Potassium-sparing diuretics (amiloride, spironolactone) act in the cortical collecting tubule where Na reabsorption is mediated by aldosterone-sensitive channels. Blockage of these channels results in a weak natriuretic activity and, due to a change in the electrical gradient, K is reabsorbed.
- Anti-diuretic hormone – ADH acts by increasing the water permeability of renal tubules, promoting water reabsorption and thus regulating the renal capacity of concentration/dilution. ADH can be released in excess (inappropriate to serum osmolality or intravascular volume) resulting in a decrease in free water excretion and hyponatremia. The syndrome of inappropriate ADH secretion (SIADH) is frequently associated with pathologies requiring intensive care management (Table 9.4), positive pressure ventilation, and various drugs. Conversely, a decrease in ADH secretion or resistance to ADH action (central or nephrogenic diabetes insipidus respectively) increases free water loss and results in the development of hypernatremia. Etiologies leading to diabetes insipidus are also common in the critical care setting (Table 9.4).

Potassium concentration regulation

K is mainly an intracellular cation (98% of total body store). Thus, small decreases in extracellular K concentration may represent a large deficit. Because of its intracellular location, K homeostasis embodies, in addition to the balance between intake and output, a rapid buffer system. This system allows rapid changes in the repartition of K between intracellular and extracellular compartments until renal elimination allows a definitive correction. Two clinically relevant systems participate in this transcellular shift:

- The Na/K ATPase system and K channels – Na/K ATPase exchange may be activated (entry of K, exit of Na) by insulin or β_2 receptor agonists, leading to a decrease in serum K concentration, or may be inhibited by digoxin.

- Exit of K from the cells may be activated by extracellular acid-base dysbalance (non-organic metabolic acidosis) or by extracellular hyperosmolality – Metabolic acidosis results in increased K exit in exchange for H^+ ions. These mechanisms of transcellular shift are cornerstones in the acute management of the dreaded hyperkalemia.

The kidneys play a major role in the maintenance of K balance in regulating the secretion of K. Relevant mechanisms implicated in the secretion/reabsorption of K include: (a) renal secretion of K directly follows serum K concentration, allowing rapid adaptation to various intakes, (b) aldosterone increases the secretion of K in the distal nephron, and (c) the secretion of K follows the flow rate in the distal nephron. Thus, increased flow (e.g., diuretics, osmotic diuresis, diabetes insipidus) results in higher K secretion (hypokalemia) while a decrease in distal flow rate (hypovolemia) results in a decrease in K secretion (hyperkalemia), and (d) to maintain electro-neutrality, the presence of anions in the distal nephron (i.e., ketones, bicarbonate) will increase the secretion of K.

Regulation of concentration of other electrolytes

Ca is mainly stored in bone. Ionized Ca is essential to muscular contraction (myocardial, smooth, skeletal), and nerve and myocardial electrical conduction. Its regulation implies intestinal absorption mediated by 1,25-dihydroxycholecalciferol, bone release of Ca stores by parathyroid hormone, and 1,25-dihydroxycholecalciferol and renal excretion, which can be increased by loop diuretics. In clinical practice it is important to consider ionized Ca or corrected Ca (which reflects the quantity of albumin which binds Ca). Mg is mainly intracellular (bone). The regulation of body stores is determined by intestinal absorption and renal excretion, influenced by diuretics (loop diuretics and thiazides) and by hypercalcemia (trans-membrane transport competition). PO_4 is the major intracellular anion and plays a critical part in energy metabolism (ATP). Estimation of PO_4 content may be difficult because of its predominantly intracellular location, rapid trans-membrane shifts, and diurnal variations in serum concentration. PO_4 is regulated by intestinal adsorption (increased by vitamin D), cellular utilization (resulting in rapid and large transcellular shifts), and mainly by renal excretion, inhibited by parathyroid hormone.

Effective hemodynamic fluid volume

Intravascular fluid volume is an important determinant of cardiac output and, depending on vascular compliance, arterial pressure. Intravascular fluid volume, along with the venous compliance, conductance and heart function, contributes to venous return and defines ventricular preload. Preload, or the stretching of myocytes at the end of diastole, is related to stroke volume (SV) by the Frank–Starling law. Heart function curves can be separated as preload dependent (the ascending part of the curve, where SV will increase following a raise in preload) or preload independent (the flat part of the curve, where SV will not increase following a raise in preload). The patient will thus be defined as fluid responder (increase in cardiac output ≥ 15% after a fluid loading) or fluid non-responder. Macro-hemodynamically speaking, patients only need fluid if the cardiac output seems inadequate for organ perfusion and if the patient is fluid responsive. Inadequate fluid infusion may induce complications (pulmonary edema, general tissue edema) and perturbations of body fluid composition (e.g. hypernatremia, hyperchloremic acidosis).

To assess hemodynamic fluid needs, clinicians must integrate indexes of preload (central venous pressure [CVP], pulmonary artery occlusion pressure [PAOP], cardiac chamber dimensions, volumetric indices), dynamic indices of preload responsiveness (stroke volume variation [SVV], pulse pressure variation [PPV]), fluid challenge tests and indices of fluid overload (clinical or radiological, extravascular lung water [EVLW]).

Static measurements of pressure (CVP, PAOP) are not good parameters of preload and do not allow fluid responsiveness to be reliably predicted. Left ventricular end-diastolic area and volumetric indexes (right ventricular end-diastolic volume and global end-diastolic volume index) perform better.

Dynamic parameters are more reliable in prediction of fluid responsiveness (preload dependency) but require specific conditions. Measurement of these indexes is based on the influence of heart–lung interaction on hemodynamics. During inspiration in positive pressure ventilation, the increase in lung volume and associated pleural pressure limits the right ventricular ejection and decreases the venous return. Consequently, left ventricular stroke volume decreases at the end of inspiration and increases at end expiration (SVV). Pulse pressure (PP = difference between systolic and diastolic blood pressure) varies according to the respiration and defines the pulse pressure variation:

$$PPV = (PPmax - PPmin) / ([PPmax + PPmin] / 2) \times 100$$

Finally, a fluid challenge (increase in cardiac output following a raise in preload) may be realized using a rapid infusion of fluid or by the passive leg raising test (PLR). PLR (45 degree from horizontal position) induces a shift of blood from the lower limbs and thus an increased cardiac preload.

Management of fluid and electrolytes in critical care

The following aspects need to be considered:
- Preset goal to define a target of fluid volumes (quantity and repartition in the different spaces) and fluid quality (including free water and electrolyte quantity and concentration) to be achieved.
- Compensation of "normal" daily fluid and electrolyte losses
  - Fluid: 30–35 mL/kg/day; 60 mL + 1 mL/kg/hour
  - Na: 1–2 mEq/kg/day
  - K: 1–1.5 mEq/kg/day
- Additional fluid or electrolyte loss/intake: must be balanced to compensate the composition of the fluids lost.

- Adaptation of the intravascular fluid volume according to the hemodynamic needs.
- Correction of the body fluid composition according to the pathophysiological mechanism.
- Monitoring of the adequacy of the body fluid (quantity and quality).

Correction of body fluid composition

Reduced total body water

Is often, but not always, associated with hypernatremia. The management consists in the correction of the underlying disease (ADH for example in diabetes insipidus) and in the replacement of body water by i.v. solutions or, if possible, by p.o. rehydration. The cumulative fluid balance does not seem suitable for monitoring the total body water; clinical examination, Na concentration, and daily body weight may be more helpful.

Increased total body water

Although the total body water is often increased in critically ill patients (third space, capillary leak) the effective hemodynamic fluid volume may be normal or even low. The management ranges from the treatment of the underlying disease to fluid restriction or administration of diuretics. For monitoring the changes the above-mentioned principles should be applied.

Hypernatremia

Hypernatremia is frequently associated with inappropriate compensation of free water loss or excessive intake of Na, in addition to a concomitant decrease in urine concentration (Table 9.4). The management consists in the correction of the underlying disorder and the compensation of the water deficit:

$$\text{Free water deficit} = 0.5 \times (\text{lean body weight [kg]}) \\ \times (\text{plasma Na [mmol/L]} / 140) - 1$$

In cases of intravascular hypovolemia, isotonic fluids are initially used (NaCl 0.9%). For other situations hypotonic fluids are preferred. The rate of correction must be calculated and, in chronic hypernatremia, must not exceed 0.5 mmol/L/h to avoid cerebral edema and intracranial hypertension.

Hyponatremia

Hyponatremia is frequently related to an impaired capacity of renal water excretion (Table 9.3). The management consists in the correction of both the underlying disorder and hypo-osmolality. Therapy includes saline infusion in situations associated with intravascular hypovolemia or a combination of water restriction and Na supplementation in case of SIADH or congestive heart failure. The rate of correction is determined by the clinical presentation but should not exceed 0.3–0.5 mmol/L/hour (too rapid correction may lead to intracellular dehydration).

In emergency situations, correction may be increased to 1 mmol/L/hour until cessation of life-threatening complications.

Hyperkalemia

Hyperkalemia may result in ECG changes and life-threatening cardiac arrhythmias. The management of hyperkalemia combines the correction of the underlying cause with reduction of K excess, according to its magnitude and clinical repercussion:

- Membrane stabilization
  - Calcium chloride/calcium gluconate
- Transcellular shift of K into the cells – temporary effect, must be associated with a definitive reduction of K excess (rebound hyperkalemia)
  - Insulin + glucose (e.g., 200 mL of glucose 20% with 15–20 IU insulin in 20–30 minutes)
  - Beta 2 agonists (salbutamol)
  - Bicarbonates (correction of concurrent metabolic acidosis)
- Increase K elimination
  - Assure renal function
  - Increase urine flow rate in the distal nephron
  - Hemodialysis
- Decrease K absorption through gastrointestinal binding of K.

Hypokalemia

Severe hypokalemia may result in various ECG changes and cardiac arrhythmias. Of particular concern in this situation is digoxin toxicity (decreases K concentration and blockage of cellular Na/K ATPase pump). In the refeeding syndrome fatal hypokalemia may occur. The management consists in the treatment of the underlying disorder together with K supplementation. Large quantities of K are often required to correct body store deficits even if the decrease in serum K is small. Intravenous infusion must be at a low rate to avoid ventricular arrhythmias (ventricular fibrillation) and through central veins (thrombophlebitis). K should not be added in dextrose solutions, which may paradoxically (due to insulin secretion) decrease K concentration. A deficit in magnesium may maintain hypokalemia and must also be corrected.

Other electrolytes

Hypercalcemia may induce hypovolemic hypernatremia (nephrogenic diabetes insipidus), vasoplegia, cardiac arrhythmias, and shock. The initial treatment of severe hypercalcemia, in addition to the treatment of the underlying disease, includes the correction of intravascular hypovolemia, hemodilution, increased excretion (furosemide, hemodialysis), and decreased bone resorption (calcitonin, bisphosphonates). The cardiotoxic effect may be antagonized by calcium channel blockers. The administration of steroids is debated.

Hypocalcemia may induce muscular spasm (Trousseau's and Chvostek's signs), vasoplegia, and cardiac arrhythmias. Treatment includes intravenous or oral (preferred) supplementation of Ca and concurrent hypomagnesemia correction. During supplementation, care must be taken in case of concurrent digoxin treatment and hyperphosphatemia (risk of calcium phosphate precipitation if $[Ca]_{serum}$ mmol $\times [P]_{serum}$ mmol > 5).

Hypomagnesemia is frequent ($> 50\%$ ICU patients) and may be associated with cardiac arrhythmias (torsades de pointes), seizures, and neuromuscular symptoms (Trousseau's sign, tetany). The management consists of Mg supplementation.

Hypermagnesemia is encountered in patients with renal failure and induced by excessive administration. In severe cases it is associated with muscle paralysis, heart conduction disturbance, and cardiac arrest. Mg is part of the treatment of various diseases encountered in critically ill patients (eclampsia, severe acute asthma). Toxicity may be partly reversed by calcium infusion, but elimination requires an increase in renal excretion.

Hypophosphatemia decreases myocardial inotropy, induces muscular weakness (delayed ventilation weaning), hemolysis, seizures, and coma. It may be encountered especially during re-nutrition of the malnourished patient (life-threatening refeeding syndrome) as well as during treatment of diabetic ketoacidosis, severe burns, or continuous hemofiltration. The management consists of PO_4 supplementation, i.v. in severe and p.o. in mild cases. Clinicians must take care of renal failure (rapid increase in PO_4 concentration) and must monitor Ca concentration (risk of hypocalcemia).

Hyperphosphatemia may induce severe hypocalcemia. The management consists of, along with treatment of the underlying disorder, enhancing renal excretion or hemodialysis.

Management of effective hemodynamic fluid volume

In situations compatible with a decrease in organ perfusion, including arterial hypotension, inadequately low cardiac output, lactic acidosis, decrease in SvO_2, and organ dysfunction (e.g., oliguria, mottled skin), we should:

- Evaluate preload
  - Very low or high CVP (lowest or highest values)
  - Very low or high PAOP (lowest or highest values)
  - Left ventricular end-diastolic areas (echocardiography)
  - Right ventricular end-diastolic volume (dedicated pulmonary artery catheter)
  - Intra-thoracic blood volume index (ITBV), global end-diastolic volume index (GEDV) (trans-pulmonary thermodilution method)
- Predict fluid responsiveness
  - PPV (probable fluid responsiveness if $> 10–17\%$)
  - SVV (probable fluid responsiveness if $> 9.5–12.5\%$)
- Fluid challenge testing
  - Improvement of cardiac output after a PLR test
  - Fluid challenge test: increase of cardiac output after infusion of a small quantity of fluid

- Consider indexes of fluid overload
  - Extravascular lung water (EVLW)
  - Radiological indices (lung edema)
  - Clinical indices (tissue edema)

Clinicians should integrate these indexes in order to determine the need and to predict the effect of fluid infusion. Fluid responsiveness alone does not *a priori* imply that a patient should receive fluids. Clinicians may use isotonic solutions with balanced electrolyte composition. Intravascular fluid volume reduction using diuretics or reducing the compensation of fluid losses may induce significant changes in body fluid composition. The discussion about the type of fluids (colloids vs crystalloids) is still ongoing and crystalloids are often preferred.

Summary points

- Fluid and electrolyte management in critical care is complex due to alterations in absorption, excretion, and distribution, as well as perturbation of hormonal state and homeostatic process by the pathology or by the treatment needed.
- Daily loss of water and electrolytes must be replaced with solutions of similar composition to the lost fluid and this replacement must be assessed with regular laboratory controls.
- Na is the primary determinant of serum osmolality. Perturbation of Na concentration (true hyper- or hyponatremia) is generally associated with similar changes in serum osmolality.
- K is mainly an intracellular cation (98% of total body store). Thus, small decreases in extracellular K concentration may represent a large deficit. The kidneys play a major role in the maintenance of K balance in regulating the secretion of K.
- The management of fluid and electrolytes in critical care needs to take into consideration: (1) definition of fluid volume and quality, (2) compensation of normal and pathological daily fluid and electrolyte losses, (3) monitoring of hemodynamic needs and adjustment of fluid volume accordingly, and (4) the pathophysiological mechanisms for the correction of the body fluid mechanisms.

Further reading

Androgué HJ, Madia NE. Hypernatremia. New Engl J Med 2000;342:1493–1499.

Androgué HJ, Madia NE. Hyponatremia. New Engl J Med 2000;342:1581–1589.

Bendjelid K. Fluid responsiveness in mechanically ventilated patients: a review of indexes used in intensive care. Crit Care Med 2003;29:352–360.

Feihl F. Interactions between respiration and systemic hemodynamics. Part I: basic concepts. Intensive Care Med 2009;35:45–54.

Feihl F. Interactions between respiration and systemic hemodynamics. Part II: practical implications in critical care. Intensive Care Med 2009;35:198–205.

Kasper DL. *Harrisson's Principles of Internal Medicine*, 16th ed. New York: McGraw-Hill; 2005.

Perren A, Markmann M, Merlani G, Marone C, Merlani P. Fluid balance in critically ill patients: should we really rely on it? Minerva Anestesiol 2011;77:802–811.

Rose BD. *Clinical Physiology of Acid-Base and Electrolyte Disorders*, 5th ed. New York: McGraw-Hill; 2001.

10

Hormonal responses and nutritional management of adults in critical care units

John A. Tayek

Metabolic changes in patients with infection, injury, or inflammatory illnesses

In patients with injury, infection, cancer, or inflammatory processes an increased blood glucose concentration is one of the most commonly observed abnormalities. This may be due to having underlying diabetes, which occurs in approximately 8% of the US population, metabolic syndrome with insulin resistance and/or pre-diabetes, which occurs in up to 30% of the US population, or due to severe injury in those without the metabolic risk for hyperglycemia. This section discusses the metabolic abnormalities in glucose, protein, and fat metabolism in this population. Specific nutritional treatment plans and considerations are also presented.

Glucose utilization in injury and infection

Glucose utilization is usually reduced in nearly all studies of glucose metabolism in patients with infection, injury, or cancer. This occurs even when the insulin concentrations are in the physiological range. This effect is not overcome even with administration of supra-physiological insulin concentrations. In sepsis, the insulin resistance associated with injury is due to defective insulin-mediated activation of the glycogen storage pathway. By approximately 7 hours after the onset of injury, there is a reduction in glucose utilization via the non-oxidative pathway. This injury response persists until the source of injury, infection, or tumor is removed.

Hepatic glucose metabolism

During infection, cancer, injury, and inflammatory illnesses, the liver increases glucose production to defend against hypoglycemia. In fact, the increase in hepatic

Nutrition in Critical Care, ed. Peter Faber and Mario Siervo. Published by Cambridge University Press. © Cambridge University Press 2014.

glucose production is the major reason why patients in the ICU have an elevated blood glucose concentration. Approximately 75% of cancer patients, like patients with infection, also have an elevated rate of glucose production. Cancer patients also have a mild form of injury, as demonstrated by mild elevation in AM serum cortisol concentration and rate of hepatic glucose production. In 18 studies, hepatic glucose production for normal volunteers ranged between 1.6 and 3.0 mg/kg/minute, with an average of 2.1 mg/kg/minute. Glucose production for cancer patients without weight loss ranged from 1.7 to 5.1 mg/kg/minute, with a mean of 2.75 mg/kg/minute. This is a 30% increase in the fasting rate of hepatic glucose production. For cancer patients with weight loss, glucose production ranged from 2.3 to 3.3 mg/kg/minute, with a mean of 2.96 mg/kg/minute. This represents a 41% increase in the rate of hepatic glucose production. Not all cancer types have an elevation in hepatic glucose production. For example, head and neck cancer patients may not have an elevation in fasting hepatic glucose production, but it is commonly elevated in lung cancer patients, probably because they have an increased injury response. The tumor burden, the cytokine and counter-regulatory hormone response, and the level of insulin resistance all play a vital role in determining the fasting blood glucose concentration in the ICU.

In cancer patients, the etiology for the elevated rate of fasting hepatic glucose production is not known. Early studies tested whether excessive growth hormone (GH) release in cancer patients might be responsible. However, there was no direct correlation between GH secretion pattern and hepatic glucose production. Koea and Shaw suggested that the rate is related to the bulk of the tumor, and others have suggested it is related to cytokines or other factors. Earlier studies on normal volunteers demonstrated that the loss of the first-phase insulin response causes a delay in the normal inhibition of glucose production. Although the latter effect may explain postprandial hyperglycemia, which is especially seen in patients with type 2 diabetes mellitus, it is an unlikely explanation for fasting hepatic glucose production.

Gluconeogenesis is elevated in head and neck cancer patients and also in lung cancer patients. Gluconeogenesis accounts for approximately 50% of the overall glucose production after an overnight fast. In 70% of published studies, cancer patients have a significant elevation in the rate of gluconeogenesis compared to normal weight-matched controls. Gluconeogenesis was directly related to the morning blood cortisol concentration in both the normal volunteers ($r = 0.913$, $p < 0.01$) and the cancer patients ($r = 0.595$, $p < 0.05$). In the septic host, the increase in glucose production is likely due to an elevation of multiple counter-regulatory hormones (cortisol, GH, catecholamines, and glucagon) and cytokines (interleukin-1 (IL-1), tumor necrosis factor-α (TNF-α), etc.).

It is important to note that unlike diabetic patients with an elevated blood glucose concentration, cancer patients with an elevated glucose production rate frequently have a normal blood glucose concentration. Fasting glucose concentrations may be 110–120 mg/dL, which may be overlooked as a subtle indicator of an elevated glucose production rate. The increased rate may contribute to an increased energy cost. Data indicate that the resting energy expenditure is elevated

Table 10.1 Mean blood glucose concentrations, hospital mortality

Patients	Controls		i.v. insulin		Reference
	Glucose (mg/dL)	Mortality (%)	Glucose (mg/dL)	Mortality (%)	
1600 mixed ICU	152	20.9	131	14.8*	Krinsley (2004)
1548 C-T surgery	153	10.9	103	7.2*	Van den Berghe et al. (2001)
139 DM with acute MI	162	26.1	153	18.6*	Malmeberg et al. (1995)
620 DM with acute MI	162	43.9	148	33.3*	Malmeberg et al. (1999)
3554 DM with C-T surgery	213	5.3	177	2.4*	Furnary et al. (2003)
Mean ± SEM	168 ± 11	21.4 ± 6.7	142 ± 12	15.3 ± 5.3	

*$p < 0.01$ vs mortality at baseline.
DM, diabetes mellitus; MI, myocardial infarction; C-T, cardiothoracic surgery.

in lung cancer patients and those with other types of cancer compared to weight-matched controls. As expected, energy expenditure is increased in most critically ill patients a few days after admission. However, the precise measurement of energy expenditure is difficult in this setting. Early in the course of critically ill patients, one should focus on excellent blood glucose control. A total caloric intake of 20–25 kcal/kg/day should be provided to the non-thermal injured adult patient. Protein intake should be 1.5 g/kg body weight/day. This has been increased to 2.0 g/kg body weight/day in adults with acute kidney injury while they stay in the ICU as recommended by the recent critical care/ASPEN guidelines (2009).

Unlike the normal fasting blood glucose that is seen in cancer patients, patients with injury or infection most commonly have an increase in blood glucose. This has been associated with a large increase in hospital mortality (Table 10.1).

Hyperglycemia as a marker of ICU mortality may be greater in surgical patients compared to medical ICU patients. In a prospective randomized clinical trial in which intravenous insulin was provided to surgical patients, preventing the increase in blood glucose associated with injury and infection, there was significantly reduced mortality.

Unfortunately, the benefits seen early on with i.v. insulin in surgical patients have not been confirmed in hospitalized patients without surgery. In the largest and most recent study, a large group of ICU patients were randomly treated with i.v. insulin to obtain a fasting blood glucose between 80 mg/dL and 110 mg/dL or keep the blood glucose between 140 mg/dL and 180 mg/dL. Hospital mortality was significantly increased in the group of patients given the i.v. insulin who had a blood glucose goal between 80 mg/dL and 110 mg/dL. The primary outcome was 90-day mortality for these ICU patients, which was increased from 24.9% in the control arm to 27.5% in the aggressive i.v. insulin arm ($p < 0.05$). This would translate to 26 more deaths in 1000 ICU patients treated with aggressive i.v. insulin. Part of the difference may have occurred due to the fact that in the surgical study by Van den Berghe, all the patients were force-fed with TPN or enteral feeding. In the other studies tight control was compared to moderate control (blood glucose under 200 mg/dL), which may have not truly tested the hypothesis that hyperglycemia (blood glucose > 199 mg/dL) is harmful in patients with sepsis. Such a study has yet to be completed to clarify the best goals for patients with hyperglycemia.

While surgical patients appear to benefit from a reduced glucose concentration after surgery, the same benefit has not been confirmed in medical patients. Patients with known diabetes and an elevated blood glucose have a very low mortality risk and may not need to be given aggressive insulin treatment when they have moderate elevations in their blood glucose concentration outside of the setting of diabetic keto-acidosis or non-ketotic hyperosmolar condition. In comparison, the mortality risk is very high in patients with new onset hyperglycemia. It is in this author's opinion that patients with new onset hyperglycemia may benefit from semi-aggressive treatment of their elevated blood glucose resulting in blood glucose concentrations between 120 and 150 mg/dL.

Protein metabolism

Many critical care patients have serious infections which are associated with an increase in skeletal muscle catabolism and a reduction in the rate of skeletal protein synthesis, both of which contribute to a large loss of lean body mass (BM) during injury and infection. In addition to sepsis, injury and cancer are also associated with muscle wasting and malnutrition. The etiology is multifactorial, including poor dietary intake, insulin resistance, elevated resting energy expenditure, and other unknown factors. Muscle wasting is due to a combination of increased skeletal muscle protein catabolism and reduced skeletal muscle protein synthesis. In humans with renal cell cancer, the rate of muscle protein synthesis was reduced. In this cancer host, the loss of skeletal muscle appears to be due in part to reduced protein synthesis and in part to a normal rate of protein catabolism. This can occur even in the face of an adequate dietary intake. Specific areas of lean BM loss that may result in a functional impairment of the respiratory muscles include the diaphragm, heart muscle, and GI mucosa. The loss of lean BM in these areas can contribute to the development of respiratory failure, heart failure, and diarrhea, respectively. The rapid development of malnutrition can occur in patients with infection due to large losses of lean BM per day.

Measurements of protein metabolism in tumor tissue have demonstrated that the tissue has a very high fractional protein synthesis rate of 50–90% per day. This is similar to that of the liver, and it contrasts with a rate of 1–3% for the skeletal muscle. However, since the body is composed mostly of skeletal muscle, its overall contribution to whole-body amino acid metabolism is large and it contributes to a significant proportion of plasma amino acid appearance rates. Data suggest that the increase in the protein catabolism in humans is via the effect of cytokines (IL-1, IL-6, and TNF) and the glucocorticoids, which are known to stimulate the ubiquitin–proteasome pathway of skeletal muscle protein catabolism. Earlier work demonstrates that TNF administration reduces skeletal muscle amino acid content by 20%, but it has no effect on skeletal muscle protein synthesis. The loss of amino acids without stimulation of protein synthesis suggests that TNF stimulates protein catabolism via a loss of amino acids from inside the skeletal muscle. This effect of TNF wanes after 6 hours since animals studied at 60 hours have a 30% increase in the rate of protein synthesis and a normal skeletal muscle amino acid content. The increased rate of protein synthesis probably reflects the recovery of the depleted amino acid pool due to earlier administration of TNF. An increase in the thyroid hormone triiodothyronine also plays an important role in promoting protein breakdown in both the ubiquitin–proteasome pathway and the lysomal pathway. However, under most conditions, patients with malignancy have either a normal or a reduced triiodothyronine concentration. Similar processes are responsible for the loss of protein seen in infection.

Data suggest that humans make and break down approximately 300 g of protein per day, which is exchanged and reused. This is mediated by the flow of amino acids into and out of cells. Since the amino acid pool is small (only 60 g), the turnover is large. Cancer patients with an elevated plasma amino acid appearance rate survive and those with a normal rate have a worse survival. In one study, stage D colorectal cancer patients who were able to sustain an increased whole-body protein metabolism over a 3-month period, as measured by amino acid kinetics, survived and those who had a normal or reduced rate died. Although fasting plasma glucose concentrations were greater in the survivors (100 ± 2 vs 92 ± 3 mg/dL), there was no difference in glucose production rate, age, and body weight. Carcino-embryonic antigen (CEA) concentrations were higher in the patients who died, which suggests that they had a larger tumor burden. There may be subgroups of patients who are able to mount an acute phase response, which may improve survival. It is not known why some patients mount an increased amino acid appearance rate with cancer, and further research is needed to confirm that it may predict survival. Historically, an elevated plasma amino acid appearance rate was believed to represent protein wasting, but recent data suggest that an elevated rate of whole-body protein metabolism may not reflect a maladaptive process but rather a healthy response to the tumor. An adequate acute phase response to tumor may reflect a greater fight against cancer. The absence of a response may be unfortunate, as data from patients with colorectal carcinoma suggest. Unfortunately, there are no similar data from infected patients for this comparison.

Lipid metabolism

Energy in the body is stored mainly in body fat, which is depleted during the wasting process. This process is normally increased during fasting without tumor or injury. When the patient has a tumor, infection, or inflammatory illness, there is a metabolic response to the injury that also promotes lipid mobilization. Several authors have implicated a lipid mobilization factor as being responsible for this process, which is believed to occur in both infection and cancer. Data suggest that this factor may also be responsible for the depletion of liver glycogen in cancer cachexia. This factor(s) increases lipolysis and plasma triglyceride concentrations. The former effect may be due to an increase in the hormone-sensitive lipase and the latter effect due to inhibition of lipoprotein lipase activity. However, the exact factor(s) that is responsible for these effects is not known. Cancer patients with weight loss have an increase in whole-body lipid turnover measured by radio-actively labeled fatty acids. However, when weight loss is prevented, there is no increase in the rate of lipolysis. Similarly, the rates of lipid oxidation are normal in cancer patients compared to weight-matched controls. In more severe injury, as seen in sepsis, the rate of lipolysis is increased.

Hormonal response to injury, infection, and cancer

Infection, cancer, or any injury to the body results in an increase in counter-regulatory hormones as well as insulin concentration. As a result of sepsis, cancer, injury, or inflammatory illnesses many patients develop the syndrome of insulin resistance even though they had no history of diabetes. In cancer patients, when the overall injury can be small, many studies have failed to demonstrate an elevation in counter-regulatory hormones. Mild elevations in cortisol concentrations may contribute to the increased protein catabolism and increased gluconeo-genesis. When serum insulin is measured with a sensitive assay, cancer patients demonstrate a small but significant elevation in serum insulin concentration. This is consistent with the observation that these patients have insulin resistance. Cancer patients, like patients with diabetes, have a reduced glucose utilization and loss of the first-phase insulin response, and many have an increased fasting hepatic glucose production rate. As mentioned previously, underweight cancer patients frequently have increased fatty acid oxidation and plasma fatty acid appearance rates. Triglyceride hydrolysis involves much more than fat oxidation, so albumin-bound fatty acids are used partially for energy but many are utilized for re-esterification or substrate cycling back to triglyceride. Similar changes in fasting insulin levels are seen in sepsis, injury, and inflammatory diseases, which also reflect a state of insulin resistance.

The rise in serum cortisol as the host's response to the tumor, injury, infection, or inflammatory illnesses is one of many factors that are responsible for the development of insulin resistance. Insulin resistance is easy to diagnose because the patient's fasting glucose will be elevated. An elevated fasting glucose level of approximately 110 mg/dL is a good marker of insulin resistance. This is not usually seen in mild injury alone unless the patient has a predisposition to the develop-ment of diabetes mellitus. Although insulin resistance is present, the presence of frank diabetes (blood glucose level > 126 mg/dL or > 7 mmol/L) is not common in cancer or mild injury. It is more common in patients with severe infection or injury. Although most of the counter-regulatory hormones are usually normal, serum cortisol and/or glucagon can be mildly elevated. Newer glucagon assays measure the normal value as 35–45 ng/mL, so a significant increase in injury can be detected, which was difficult to do with the older glucagon assays. Data from pancreatic cancer patients have shown elevated glucagon concentrations, which may be contributing to the development of diabetes. Earlier work found that GH secretion was increased in cancer patients by 24-hour analysis and by random sampling. However, after careful study, the increase in GH does not appear to have a major influence on hepatic glucose metabolism. Although there may be a small effect on glycogen breakdown, the major effect is likely via inhibition of glucose utilization in the skeletal muscle.

The sick euthyroid state, in which total triiodothyronine (T3) concentrations are reduced in severely injured and infected patients, is common. This is likely a normal response to conserve energy in the injured person as the body's ability to convert the stored form of a thyroid hormone (thyroxine (T4)) into the active form of thyroid hormone, T3, becomes impaired. T4 is converted to an inactive thyroid hormone known as reverse-T3 hormone (rT3). This event may have evolved as a necessary energy-saving response during a severe injury or illness to reduce the known contribution of T3 to resting energy expenditure. The low T3 syndrome is an adaptive way to reduce the normal day-to-day effect of T3 on resting energy expenditure. This process can occur in the aggressive cancers, for which the patient's response is similar to that of an injury response.

In septic and injured patients, all counter-regulatory hormones are routinely elevated, contributing to an increase in protein catabolism, glucose production, gluconeogenesis, and glycogen breakdown and a major reduction in glucose utilization and anabolism.

The ABCD score: an acute predictor of hospital survival in patients with infection, injury, or inflammation

New onset hyperglycemia in non-diabetic patients (fasting blood glucose > 125 mg/dL or non-fasting > 199 mg/dL) increases hospital mortality by 4- to 20-fold. While having an elevated blood glucose associated with diabetes appears to have risk, the risk associated with not having diabetes and an elevated blood glucose is dramatic. As mentioned above the amount of weight loss upon presentation to hospital predicts hospital outcome. In addition, the serum albumin concentration also predicts hospital mortality. Lastly, calorie intake in the hospital predicts hospital outcome. To simplify the estimate of mortality risk in the hospital an ABCD score for hospital outcome was developed. The score consists of adding points to mortality risk based on serum albumin, weight loss, and calorie intake (See Table 10.2). All values can be collected over a single day. If the patients are put NPO they should receive no points for calorie intake but if they chose not to eat then the amount eaten is calculated into their ABCD score. Each component

Table 10.2 ABCD Score for Hospital Mortality (Albumin, Body Weight, Calorie Intake and New Onset Hyperglycemia (looks like Diabetes))

Clinical variable	Change	Score
Reduced serum albumin	< 3.0 g/dL minimal	5
	< 2.5 g/dL mild	10
	< 2.0 g/dL moderate	20
	< 1.5 g/dL severe	30
	< 1.0 g/dL dangerous	40
Weight loss	≥ 10% mild or BMI < 22	5
	> 20% moderate or BMI < 20	10
	≥ 30% severe or BMI < 18	15
Calorie intake	< 50% of goal (< 1000 calories)	2
	< 25% of goal (< 500 calories)	4
	Zero calorie intake	6
New onset hyperglycemia FBG > 125 mg/dL × 2 (or non-fasting glucose > 199 mg/dL × 2; or one each; do not include known diabetic patients)	2-fold	

Add up risk to obtain hospital mortality risk. If new onset hyperglycemia, multiply the risk by two.

For example, 30 points represents a 30% mortality rate risk, 60 points a 60% mortality rate risk, and 100 points a 100% mortality rate risk.

(serum albumin, weight loss, and calorie intake) of the ABCD score is independently associated with risk of mortality, which can be minimized by accurate diagnostic protocols and appropriate nutritional interventions.

Nutritional feeding: enteral versus parenteral

In all situations, if the gut is functional, then it should be used as the route of calorie administration. Gut atrophy predisposes to bacterial and fungal colonization and subsequent invasion associated with bacteremia. Recent data demonstrated that TPN should only be given to critically ill non-severely malnourished patients after 8 days of ICU stay. Patients who received TPN early had a higher infection rate (26.2 vs 22.8%, $p < 0.05$), more patients requiring more than 2 days of mechanical ventilation, and a 3-day increase in the need for renal replacement therapy.

Enteral products

Enteral nutrition is best taken by mouth if the patient can ingest the required amount. If the patient cannot, then either supplements or full tube feeding is the method of choice. Protein in the peptide form is better absorbed than the free amino acid form due to specific transporters in the small intestines for amino acids, dipeptides, and tripeptides. Feeding tube placement is best in the small bowel up to the ligament of Treitz. The infusion of enteral products into the small bowel will reduce the incidence of aspiration because the infusion is below the pylorus. Intubated patients have a low risk for aspiration due to the endotracheal cuff, so placement of a feeding tube into the small bowel is less essential.

Supplementation of enteral products with higher than standard amounts of the amino acid arginine has been done to enhance immune function. Published data on its beneficial effect in surgical patients have demonstrated some benefit; however, data from non-surgical patients suggest harm. Immunonutrition should not be given to patients with severe infection, especially patients with pneumonia.

Branched-chain amino acid-enriched enteral products are available and have been shown to improve mental function and mortality in patients with hepatic encephalopathy. Albumin synthesis is also stimulated by branched-chain-enriched amino acid solutions. However, additional branched-chain amino acids did not improve morbidity or mortality in trauma or septic patients randomized to receive branched-chain-enriched amino acids compared to conventional feeding. Glutamine-enriched enteral formulas are very common. There are many enteral products used in hospitalized patients and for home enteral nutritional support.

The choice of lipid composition in enteral products is a field that is rapidly evolving, and this is an important decision to be made by the clinician depending on the type of disease being treated. The use of omega-3-enriched fatty acids in the enteral product (fish oil-enriched) has been associated with an ability to modify the inflammatory response that may be related to the increased arachidonic acid metabolism and a decrease in the omega-6 pathway fatty acid metabolism. Unfortunately, most commercially available enteral products that have omega-3 fatty acids also have other additives, such as arginine, glutamine, and nucleotides, so that the benefits attributed to the use of an omega-3-enriched fatty acid enteral diet await future clinical studies.

Energy intake

Elderly hospitalized patients who consume less than 50% of their estimated maintenance caloric requirement have an 8-fold increase in hospital mortality (11.8 vs 1.5%). This suggests that an intake of less than 1000 kcal may not be helpful. In a prospective study providing approximately 400 additional calories as "sip feeds," reduced mortality was seen in severely malnourished (BMI < 5th percentile), medically ill elderly patients. In this study, patients were randomized to receive 120 mL of enteral supplements provided by the registered nurse three times per day or provided no additional sip feeds. Patients who received the sip feeds had a significantly better energy intake (1409 kcal) than non-supplemented patients (1090 kcal), and they had an increased overall weight gain compared with a loss in the controls. Patients in the underweight group who received intervention had a significant reduction in mortality compared to controls (15 vs 35%, $p < 0.05$).

In the third study, patients with less than 25% of recommended calorie intake (< 600 kcal) had a 3.7-fold increased rate of nosocomial bloodstream infections. The energy intake is a surrogate marker of protein intake in the critically ill. Usually the protein content of food and enteral products given to critically ill patients is 20%. There are also data that suggest hypocaloric feeding in the critically ill where protein intake is provided at the required level can improve outcome in certain circumstances. Protein intake, in this author's opinion, is more important than total calorie intake. This is especially true if the calorie intake results in new onset hyperglycemia, which can be seen in many critically ill patients who have a history of pre-diabetes (HbA1c of 5.7 to 6.4%).

Summary points

- Hyperglycemia is one of the most common metabolic abnormalities in patients with infectious, traumatic, and inflammatory illnesses. This is mostly related to a reduced glucose utilization and increased hepatic gluconeogenesis.
- Hyperglycemia appeared to be associated with an increased risk of ICU mortality. However, while surgical patients appear to benefit from a reduced glucose concentration after surgery, the same benefit has not been confirmed in ICU medical patients.
- An increase in counter-regulatory hormones as well as insulin concentration is observed in critically ill patients. As a result of sepsis, cancer, injury, or inflammatory illnesses many patients develop the syndrome of insulin resistance even though they had no history of diabetes.
- Critical care patients are characterized by an enhanced catabolic response and linked to protein and lipid mobilization.
- Mortality risk is high in patients with new onset hyperglycemia. Patients with new onset hyperglycemia may benefit from semi-aggressive treatment of their elevated blood glucose resulting in blood glucose concentrations between 120 and 150 mg/dL.

Further reading

Barringer TA, Kirk JK, Santaniello AC, Foley KL, Michielutte R. Effect of multivitamin and mineral supplement on infection and quality of life. Ann Inter Med 2003;138:365–371.

Carson GL. Insulin resistance in human sepsis: implications for nutritional and metabolic care of the critically ill surgical patient. Ann Royal Coll Surg 2004;86:75–81.

Caster MP, Mesotten D, Hermans G, et al. Early versus late parenteral nutrition in critically ill adults. New Engl J Med 2011;365:506–517.

Christiansen C, Tolf P, Jorgensen HS, Andersen SK, Tonnesen E. Hyperglycemia and mortality in critically ill patients. Intensive Care Med 2004;30:1685–1688.

Fawzi WW, Msamanga GI, Spiegelman D, et al. A randomized trial of multivitamin supplements and HIV disease progression and mortality. New Engl J Med 2004;35:23–32.

Furnary AP, Gao G, Grunkemeier GL, et al. Continuous insulin infusion reduces mortality in patients with diabetes undergoing coronary artery bypass grafting. J Thorac Cardiovasc Surg 2003;125(5):1007–1021.

Hiesmayr M, Schindler K, Pernicka E, et al. Decreased food intake is a risk factor for mortality in hospitalized patients: The Nutrition Day survey 2006. Clin Nutr 2009;28: 484–491.

Koea J, Shaw JFH. The effect of tumor bulk on the metabolic response to cancer. Ann Surg 1992;215:282–288.

Krinsley JS. Effect of an intensive glucose management protocol on the mortality of critically ill adult patients. Mayo Clin Proc 2004;79(8):992–1000.

Malmberg K, Rydén L, Efendic S, et al. Randomized trial of insulin-glucose infusion followed by subcutaneous insulin treatment in diabetic patients with acute myocardial infarction (DIGAMI study): effects on mortality at 1 year. J Am Coll Cardiol 1995;26 (1):57–65.

Malmberg K, Norhammar A, Wedel H, Rydén L. Glycometabolic state at admission: important risk marker of mortality in conventionally treated patients with diabetes mellitus and acute myocardial infarction: long-term results from the Diabetes and Insulin-Glucose Infusion in Acute Myocardial Infarction (DIGAMI) study. Circulation 1999;99(20):2626–2632.

McClave SA, Martindale RG, Vanek VW, et al. Guidelines for the provision and assessment of nutrition support therapy in the adult critically ill. J Parenter Enteral Nutr 2009;33;277.

Plank LD, Hill GL. Energy balance in critical illness. Proc Nutr Soc 2003;62:545–552.

Ramaswamy G, Rao VR, Kumaraswamx SV, Anantha N. Serum vitamin status in oral leucoplakia: a preliminary study. Eur J Cancer 1996;328(2):120–122.

Rubinson L, Diette GB, Song X, Grower RG, Krishnan JA. Low calorie intake is associated with nosocomial bloodstream infections in patients in the medical intensive care unit. Crit Care Med 2004;32:350–357.

Scjmeoder SM, Veyres P, Pivot X, et al. Malnutrition is an independent factor associated with nosocomial infections. Br J Nutr 2004;92:105–111.

Tayek JA. A review of cancer cachexia and abnormal glucose metabolism in humans with cancer. J Am Coll Nutr 1992;11:445–456.

Tayek JA, Brasel JA. Failure of anabolism in malnourished cancer patients receiving growth hormone. J Clin Endocrinol Metab 1995;80:2082–2087.

Tayek JA, Katz J. Glucose production, recycling, and gluconeogenesis in normals and diabetics; mass isotopomer U-13C glucose study. Am J Physiol 1996;270:E709–E717.

Tayek JA, Katz J. Glucose production, recycling, Cori cycle and gluconeogenesis in humans with and without cancer: relationship to serum cortisol concentration. Am J Physiol 1997;272:E476–E484.

Tayek CJ, Tayek JA. Diabetes patients' and non-diabetic patients' intensive care unit and hospital mortality risks associated with sepsis. World J Diabetes 2012;3:29–34.

Van den Berghe G, Wouters P, Weekers F, et al. Intensive insulin therapy in critically ill patients. New Engl J Med 2001;345:1359–1367.

Ziegler TR. Clinical and metabolic efficacy of glutamine-supplemented parenteral nutrition after bone marrow transplantation. Ann Intern Med 1992;116:821.

Nutritional Support for Specific Conditions and Pathologies

11

Nutritional support of critically ill burn patients

Bjarne F. Alsbjoern

Introduction

The metabolic response of patients with burns increases immediately after the accident. For burns covering more than 40% of the body surface area (BSA) the metabolic rate may increase by as much as 100–150%. If these requirements are not compensated for with sufficient nutritional support, an array of problems will compound the long and difficult recovery of the burns patient. The relationship between increased metabolic demands and burns injuries was first elucidated more than 60 years ago. Initially, nutrition was administered by the parenteral route. However, it was soon observed that enteral feeding protocols offered clear advantages in patient care as enteral feeding is usually simpler to establish, easier to administrate, and very importantly facilitates the preservation of the general gut function and mucosal barrier, thus minimizing the transfer of gut toxins to the blood. Additionally, enteral feeding protocols offer clear financial advantages to parenteral nutrition.

The hyper-metabolic state will continue for weeks after the injury and is proportional to: (1) the severity of the accident, (2) time of wound debridement and closure, and (3) the onset of rehabilitation. An increase in body temperature and oxygen consumption further adds to the increase in metabolic rate as does an enhanced cardiac output. These physiological effects of burn injuries all additionally contribute to the increase in energy expenditure which must overall be balanced with an increased energy intake. Total energy and macronutrient intake must be carefully considered as patients rapidly enter a state of negative nitrogen balance. Protein loss from wounds will soon be compounded by severe skeletal muscle decay. This effect of burns injury is even observed in patients receiving a high-protein diet.

Nutrition in Critical Care, ed. Peter Faber and Mario Siervo. Published by Cambridge University Press. © Cambridge University Press 2014.

To mitigate the hyper-metabolic state, patients should be nursed in rooms kept at temperatures of 25–30°C and receive high standard pain control, meticulous wound care to avoid infection, anxiolytics to reduce patient anxiety, and early surgical wound debridement and closure. Interestingly, treatment with beta-blockers has been suggested to abate the metabolic response in this group of patients.

The immediate problem contributing to the metabolic changes of the burned patient is the destruction of the epithelial layer of the skin (stratum corneum) resulting in a severe loss of fluid, protein, vitamins, and minerals.

Patients with burns of more than 15% BSA in the early period following injury are at risk of gastro-enteral paralysis. This may initially render enteral nutrition difficult to establish and staff should be vigilant and actively encourage patients to eat and drink. Importantly, a dietician should monitor the metabolic state of the patient daily and in detail plan the nutritional requirements from assessments of basal metabolic rate and increased calorific needs. Additionally, from minutes after the accident, patients sustain a compromised immune system putting them at high risk of attracting infections and aggravating the hyper-metabolic state. Antibiotics should be administered according to local protocols.

Fluid resuscitation

Children with burns of more than 10% BSA and adults with more than 15% BSA suffer from such intense water evaporation that intravenous fluids should be administered (Fig. 11.1). The most frequently used formula to calculate fluid substitution is the Parkland formula:

$$\text{Fluid for the first 24 hours(mL)}$$
$$= 4\,\text{ml} \times \text{body weight in kilograms(kg-BW)} \times \%\,\text{burned BSA.}$$

The fluid is administered as Ringer's lactate solution. Half of the calculated volume should be administered in the first 8 hours and the remaining half over 16 hours. When sufficiently rehydrated the urine output should be at least 1 mL/kg-BW/hour. The Parkland formula can induce a slight overhydration resulting in increased intra-abdominal pressure (IAP) causing splanchnic ischemia and renal impairment. Furthermore, a high IAP will reduce blood flow in the vena cavae system and splinting of the diaphragm compromising pulmonary function. Such adverse physiological effects of fluid resuscitation are currently the focus of intense research.

In addition to evaporative water loss an increased capillary permeability results in the loss of water and small proteins to the extravascular space. This effect of burns is most profound during the first 24 hours and can to a certain extent be alleviated by the administration of intravenous albumin. To guide the assessment of fluid and nutritional substitution patients with burns should be weighed daily.

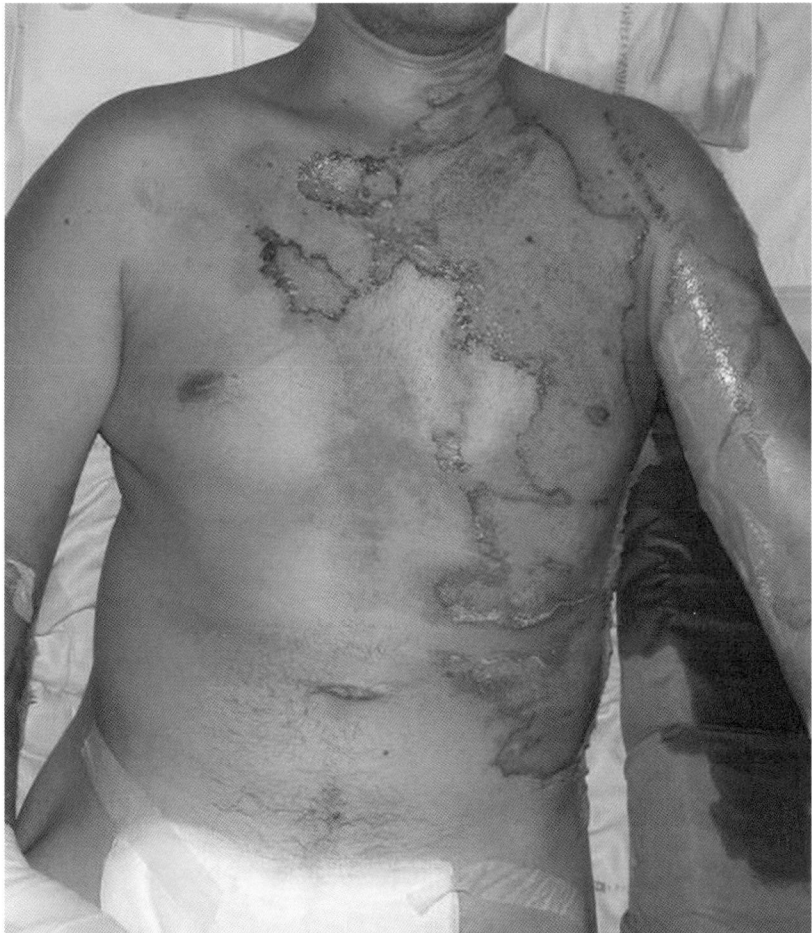

Figure 11.1 Severe fluid and protein loss from a 2nd degree burn wound.

Total energy requirements

To assess total energy requirements several formulas have been developed during the last 60 years. Ideally, energy requirements should be guided by indirect calorimetry and laboratory measurements of nitrogen balance. However, clinical restrictions rarely allow these measurements and instead the equations given below can be used for calculating daily energy requirements:

Curreri equations:

Children
    0–1 years: BMR + 63 kJ × % BSAB
    1–3 years: BMR + 105 kJ × % BSAB
    4–15 years: BMR + 167 kJ × % BSAB

Adults
16–59 years: 105 kJ /kg + 167 kJ × % BSAB
>60 years: 85 kJ /kg + 272 kJ × % BSAB

Galveston equations:

Children
0–1 years: 8778 kJ/m^2+ 4180 kJ/m^2 burn
1–11 years: 7524 kJ/m^2 + 5434 kJ/m^2 burn

Adults
6270 kJ/m^2 + 6270 kJ/m^2 burn

Copenhagen equations:

Children
0–3 years: 420 kJ/kg + 63 kJ/%BSAB
4–10 years: 315 kJ/kg + 63 kJ/%BSAB
11–15 years: 210 kJ/kg + 84 kJ/%BSAB

Adults
84 kJ/kg + 294 kJ/%BSAB

where BMR = basal metabolic rate, BSA = body surface area, %BSAB = % body surface area burned.

As indicated by the above equations the total energy requirement not only varies with the severity of the injury but also with the patient's age and body weight. Compared with adults children have a relatively higher body surface area when corrected for body weight.

Protein requirements

The exaggerated protein loss from wound exudate and nitrogen in urine increase the demands for protein intake. Increased protein turnover and loss is significant during the first 2 weeks and will then gradually settle as the patient recovers by conservative and surgical treatment. Protein requirements can be estimated by the Liljedahl formula:

	Children	Adults
Liljedahl	3g/kg + 1g/%BSAB	1g/kg + 3g/% BSAB
Copenhagen	3g/kg + 1g/%BSAB	1g/kg + 2g/% BSAB

The Copenhagen formula is used for only the first 3 days. After day 3 and until full recovery the daily protein requirements of adults are estimated from nitrogen loss calculated from urinary urea excretion. In clinical practice protein substitution is categorized upon whether total urinary urea excretion is less or more than 300 mmol/day:

Daily urinary urea excretion < 300 mmol/day:

Grams protein/day (to achieve nitrogen balance) = total urinary urea in mmol/day × 0.18 + 12.5 grams of protein

Daily urinary urea excretion > 300 mmol/day:

Grams protein/day (to achieve nitrogen balance) = total urinary urea mmol/day × 0.18 + 25 grams of protein

The factor 0.18 converts mmol urea into grams of protein. Additions of 25 and 12.5 g/day are made for protein losses from feces, skin, and miscellaneous. For children the factors 25 and 12.5 are multiplied by body weight in kilograms and divided by 70 (empirically representing the weight of an adult). As daily urinary urea loss in children rarely exceeds 300 mmol/day, the equivalent formula becomes:

Grams protein/day (to achieve nitrogen balance) = total urinary urea in mmol/day × 0.18 + 12.5 × BW/70 grams of protein

In choosing nutritional formulations and diet the ratio of calories to protein intake should be high in order to avoid protein becoming an energy source.

Lipid requirements

The increase in metabolic rate facilitates lipolysis contributing to the inevitable weight loss observed in burns patients. It is recommended that total energy intake from fat should be 25–30% for adults and up to 50% in children less than 1 year.

Carbohydrate requirements

The remaining energy requirements not met by protein and fat should be substituted by carbohydrates.

Vitamin requirements

The increase in metabolic rate also results in increased requirements for vitamins and trace elements as these constitute important parts of a scavenger system involved in reducing the blood concentration of free oxygen radicals. This is important as the blood concentration of free oxygen radicals is elevated in trauma patients further aggravating the inflammatory response.

The precise dose and time of administration remains disputed. In Copenhagen the daily supplements are:

- Children (2–12 years) with more than 10% BSA burns
- Adults with more than 40% BSA burns

Children (2–12 yrs) with more than 10% BSA burns	Adults with more than 40% BSA burns
One children's vitamin pill/drops	One multivitamin pill
Vitamin A 4500 IE	Vitamin A 9000 IE
Vitamin C 250 mg	Vitamin C 1000 mg
Vitamin B1 100 mg	Vitamin B1 900 mg
Folinic acid 0.4 mg	Folinic acid 0.4 mg
	Vitamin E 100 mg/week
Zinc 22 mg	Zinc 44 mg

Route of nutrient supplementation

Enteral feeding

When the total energy requirements and macronutrient substitution have been calculated, preferably an enteral feeding route should be established. However, after major burns constituting more than 40% BSA parenteral supplementation most often becomes necessary during the period of early treatment.

A nasogastric or nasoenteral feeding tube should be placed. The nasoenteral tube has the advantage of reducing the risk of aspiration to the airways. This is particularly important bearing in mind that gastric paralysis frequently occurs during the early days after the injury. The position of the feeding tube should be secured and checked regularly.

Enteral feeding should preferably be initiated within the first 24 hours after the injury.

Parenteral feeding

This route should be reserved for patients where enteral nutrition cannot meet the required energy intake or injuries prevent the establishment of enteral feeding.

Apart from the disadvantages to the gut function the parenteral route of nutrition carries an increased risk of local infection and sepsis in immuno-compromised patients.

Summary points

- After severe burns injury energy requirements may more than double.
- Fluid and energy resuscitation should follow published guidelines.
- Protein requirements increase significantly.
- Enteral feeding should be established at the earliest opportunity.
- Patients should receive vitamin supplementations.

Further reading

Alsbjoern B, Gilbert P, Hartmann B, et al. Guidelines for the management of partial-thickness burns in general hospital or community setting: recommendations of a European working party. Burns 2007;33:155–160.

Davies JWL, Liljedahl S. Metabolic consequences of an extensive burn. In: Polk HC, Stone HH (eds) *Contemporary Burn Management*. Boston: Little, Brown and Company; 1971:151.69.

Day T, Dean P, Adams MC, et al. Nutritional requirements of the burned child: the Curreri Junior Formula. Proc Am Burn Assoc 1986;18:86.

For de G, Jennings M, Andrassy RI. Serum albumin (oncotic pressure) correlates with enteric feeding tolerance in the pediatric surgical patient. J Pediatr Surg 1987;22:597–600.

Herndon DN, Wolf SE, Chinkes DL, Wolfe RR. Reversal of catabolism by beta-blockade after severe burns. New Engl J Med 2001;345:1223–1229.

Hildreth MA, Herndon DN, Desai MH, Broemeling LD. Current treatment reduces calories required to maintain weight in pediatric patients with burns. J Burn Care Rehabilitation 1990;11:405–409.

Pasulka PS, Wachtel TL. Nutritional considerations for the burned patient. Surg Clin North Am 1987;67:109–131.

12

Nutritional support of critically ill neurosurgical patients

Roland N. Dickerson and Peter Faber

Survivors of severe traumatic brain injury (TBI) and spinal cord injury (SCI) are potentially left with substantial cognitive and/or physical impairment. Early and adequate nutritional therapy is challenging in these patients, but if achieved, can also potentially improve clinical outcomes, particularly for the patient with TBI.

Traumatic brain injury

Clinical relevancy

Patients suffering from severe TBI (Glasgow Coma Scale <8) are among the most hyper-metabolic and hyper-catabolic of all critically ill patients, second only to those with substantial thermal injury. Since the rate of protein catabolism during the acute phase post-injury can exceed three to four times the rate of body protein loss compared to simple starvation in unstressed individuals, marked protein depletion can occur rapidly. A Cochrane analysis of nutritional support in TBI patients has concluded that early nutrition therapy reduces infection rates and may improve survival for patients. Most clinicians therefore view early and adequate nutrition therapy as essential for achievement of a positive clinical outcome. Early nutrition therapy may be defined as initiation of therapy within 24 to 72 hours of injury. However, most of the studies examining early versus delayed nutrition therapy used the definition of early nutrition therapy as within 48 hours of injury.

Enteral versus parenteral nutrition and gastric feeding intolerance

Most of the studies showing improved clinical benefit from early nutrition therapy for patients with TBI utilized PN as the predominant source of protein and calories as patients were considered to be intolerant to early EN. Slowed gastric emptying has been reported in up to 30% to 50% of critically ill patients and can result in increased gastric residual volumes and gastric feeding intolerance. These data have led some clinicians to prefer small bowel feeding for these patients.

Some of the studies comparing PN to EN for patients with TBI used the non-specific "presence of bowel sounds" as a marker for readiness of the gastrointestinal

Nutrition in Critical Care, ed. Peter Faber and Mario Siervo. Published by Cambridge University Press. © Cambridge University Press 2014.

tract for feeding. Other criteria for withholding of enteral feeding in many of the older studies often employed gastric residual volumes (GRV), which are considered unacceptably low (e.g., 50 mL to 150 mL) by today's standards (e.g., 200 mL to 500 mL). The inappropriate use of these markers, lack of availability or knowledge of current prokinetic therapy, and difficulty associated with small bowel feeding tube placement may have also led to the early initiation of PN and abandonment of early EN. Thus, when the patients who received PN were compared to those who received EN, it was, realistically, a comparison of early "adequate calories and protein" versus "marginal or inadequate calories and protein." This difference in nutritional intake likely explains the benefit of early PN over early EN for patients with TBI as described in these older studies.

Our published data in 882 trauma patients (49% with TBI) indicated that patients with TBI exhibited a 19% gastric feeding intolerance rate compared to 10% of trauma patients without TBI. Thus, the incidence of clinically relevant gastric feeding tolerance for patients with TBI is probably not as prevalent as previously thought (e.g., ~50% to 80%). However, it is important to note that the rate of EN gastric feeding intolerance for trauma patients with TBI is still twice that of trauma patients without TBI. Those patients with more severe disease, as evidenced by elevated intracranial pressures (ICPs) in excess of 20 mmHg or who receive more aggressive pharmacotherapy (e.g., pentobarbital, neuromuscular blocking agents, or propofol) are also more likely to have gastric feeding intolerance.

The North American Consensus on Aspiration (2002) recommends withholding feeding for a GRV > 500 mL and initiation of an algorithmic approach to reduce risk of aspiration for patients with a GRV within 200 to 500 mL. As a result, we use a GRV of >200 mL along with a physical abdominal exam and interview of the patient for any adverse abdominal signs (e.g., distension, tympanic) or symptoms (e.g., nausea, vomiting, pain, bloating, or cramping) as evidence for gastric feeding intolerance. If the patient experiences a single elevated GRV above 200 mL without abnormal abdominal signs or any adverse symptoms of gastric feeding intolerance, the EN is continued. If the patient has an abnormal abdominal exam or experiences adverse symptoms, the feedings are temporarily withheld and initiation of prokinetic therapy is initiated.

Prokinetic therapy

In the United States, prokinetic agents for routine use in hospitalized patients are the dopamine-2 receptor antagonist metoclopramide and the motilin receptor agonist erythromycin. Recent data suggest that erythromycin is more effective than metoclopramide and additional studies indicate that combined metoclopramide-erythromycin therapy is more effective than either drug when used as monotherapy. This is particularly pertinent for TBI patients as they experience substantially more tachyphylaxis to metoclopramide monotherapy than trauma patients without TBI. Patients with a severely elevated intracranial pressure (ICP) >20 mm Hg also respond less favorably to initial therapy with metoclopramide than those with less severe ICP elevation.

The optimal dose of metoclopramide and erythromycin is conflicting. Our data indicated a success rate of 55% (45% for patients with TBI and 64% for those without TBI) for 10 mg of intravenous metoclopramide given every 6 hours and 62% (53% for TBI, 80% without TBI) for those who received 20 mg per dose. We employ intravenous erythromycin at a dose of 250 mg every 6 hours. Combined intravenous metoclopramide and erythromycin therapy achieved a success rate of 79% (78% and 80% with and without TBI, respectively). At our institution, we prefer to use therapeutic antibiotic doses of erythromycin since giving lower doses provides an environment for the induction of bacterial resistance. In addition, we have observed that tachyphylaxis over a 7-day observation period for all trauma patients is substantially reduced with combination therapy as compared to meto-clopramide monotherapy (10% versus 20% decline in efficacy, respectively). Our empirical approach to prokinetic therapy is to give metoclopramide monotherapy as first-line therapy for trauma and surgical patients without TBI. For patients with TBI, combined therapy is initially indicated.

Erythromycin for critically ill patients has some potential life-threatening complications with reports of prolongation of the Q-T interval by ∼30 to 40ms, Torsades des Points, and sudden death from cardiac causes. Additionally, erythromycin has numerous drug interactions interfering with the metabolism of other drugs that depend on the cytochrome P450 3A4 isoenzyme. Before erythromycin is given, the patient's medication profile should be reviewed for any pertinent drug interactions and a baseline Q-Tc interval obtained. If no drug interactions are present, the patient's Q-Tc interval is less than ∼425 ms, and the medical history is absent of cardiac complications requiring pharmacotherapy, erythromycin may be added to the metoclopramide therapy. Once the gastric residual volumes are negligible without any abdominal signs or symptoms of gastric feeding intolerance, erythromycin can be discontinued, followed by metoclopramide therapy on the following day as long as gastric feeding tolerance is maintained.

Estimation of energy requirements

The severity of hypermetabolism in TBI patients is variable, ranging from 90% to over 200% of predicted energy expenditure. This variability can be explained by severity of injury, muscle contractions and posturing, fever, sympathetic storming, dysautonomia, diet-induced thermogenesis, sepsis, and concurrent pharmaco-therapy. Indirect calorimetry for the measurement of energy expenditure is not readily available at most institutions and many clinicians therefore attempt to use common equations for predicting basal energy expenditure and then add a "stress factor" for injuries or "a reduction factor" for concurrent energy expenditure-reducing pharmacotherapy. However, addition of "stress factors" can easily lead to overfeeding of the critically ill patient with TBI. Improvement in sedation and analgesia is likely to account for the perceived reduction in energy requirements from the current literature as compared to older studies. For example, continuous intravenous infusion of propofol reduces cerebral metabolism and as a result reduces whole-body oxygen consumption by as much as 25% to 40%. It is also important to recognize that propofol is delivered to the patient in an intravenous 10% soybean oil emulsion which delivers 1.1 kcal/mL.

The 2007 Brain Trauma Foundation guidelines recommend a broad total caloric intake within 100% to 140% of predicted (basal) energy expenditure. The Penn State equation (example in Table 12.1) is probably the best predictive formula for estimating energy expenditure of critically ill trauma patients including those with TBI, predicting energy expenditure within 10% of measured energy expenditure 72% of the time for patients with isolated TBI and 73% of the time for patients with multiple traumatic injuries including TBI. The predictive method was unbiased and had a mean absolute error of

Table 12.1 How to use the Penn State equation*

$$REE = (\text{Mifflin} \times 0.96) + (\text{Tmax} \times 167) + (V_E \times 31) - 6212$$

Mifflin (REE in healthy subjects) equations:

Male : $(\text{Weight} \times 10) + (\text{Height} \times 6.25) - (\text{age} \times 5) + 5$
Female : $(\text{Weight} \times 10) + (\text{Height} \times 6.25) - (\text{age} \times 5) - 161$

Where REE is resting energy expenditure in kcal/d, Mifflin is the Mifflin–St. Jeor equation in kcal/d, Tmax is maximum daily temperature in °C, V_E is minute ventilation in L/min, Weight is in kg, Height is in cm.

*The Penn State formula given above should not be used for patients >60 years of age or for those whose BMI is >30 kg/m^2.

Case scenario: A 40-year-old man is admitted to the intensive care unit following a motor vehicle collision. He is noted to have multiple rib fractures and a severe TBI. He receives fentanyl and midazolam for analgesia and sedation. He is mechanically ventilated with a minute ventilation of 8 L/min. His height is 174 cm and weight 85 kg. His maximum temperature for the past 24 hours was 38.0°C. What is his estimated REE?

Step 1. Calculate the Mifflin REE

$$\begin{aligned} \text{Mifflin (kcals/d)} &= (85\,\text{kg} \times 10) + (174 \times 6.25) - (40 \times 5) + 5 \\ &= (850) + (1088) - (200) + 5 \\ &= 1743 \end{aligned}$$

Step 2. Calculate the Penn State REE

$$\begin{aligned} \text{Mifflin(kcals/d)} &= (\text{Mifflin} \times 0.96) + (\text{Tmax} \times 167) + (V_E \times 31) - 6212 \\ &= (1743 \times 0.96) + (38 \times 167) + (8 \times 31) - 6212 \\ &= 1673 + 6346 + 248 - 6212 \\ &= 2055\ (24\,\text{kcal/kg/d}) \end{aligned}$$

Step 3. Estimate caloric requirements/goal

$$\begin{aligned} \text{Caloric goal} &= \sim 1.2\ \text{to}\ 1.3 \times \text{REE} \\ &= 2466\ \text{kcals/d}\ (29\,\text{kcal/kg/d})\ \text{to}\ 2672\ \text{kcals/d}\ (31\,\text{kcal/kg/d}) \end{aligned}$$

170 + 149 kcals/day. However, the method can be somewhat tedious in that the Mifflin–St. Jeor equation for healthy adults is employed in the regression along with minute ventilation (obtained from the patient's ventilator) and maximum temperature for the day. Thus, calculations may need to be redone daily for most patients. Since the predictive method estimates resting energy expenditure and not total energy expenditure in the ICU, some clinicians will provide 10% more than predicted to account for this difference (e.g., ≤10%) as well as an additional 10% for the specific dynamic action of nutrient metabolism. Despite improved accuracy for predicting measured energy expenditure with the Penn State equation, some clinicians still prefer to use the less accurate 25 to 35 kcal/kg/day or 1.3 to 1.5 × Harris–Benedict equations. Use of estimates of energy requirements mandates close monitoring of the patient for evidence of overfeeding (e.g., increase in pCO_2 or worsened hyperglycemia).

One exception whereby the Penn State, 25 to 30 kcal/kg/d, and 1.3 to 1.5 × Harris–Benedict methods should not be used is when the patient is being given pentobarbital for an elevated ICP that is refractory to conventional therapy. Pentobarbital therapy may markedly decrease measured energy expenditure by 30% to 50%. Under these conditions, our current practice is to be very conservative with caloric intakes and not exceed 1 × Harris–Benedict equations or 20 to 25 kcal/kg/day. The Penn State equation has not been evaluated for patients with TBI receiving pentobarbital therapy.

Estimation of protein requirements

Traumatic injury is associated with a substantial increase in urinary nitrogen excretion compared to healthy subjects. Whole-body protein synthesis increases by 15% to 27% and protein breakdown increases by 41% to 79%. In our study with 83 trauma patients with TBI and 166 trauma patients without TBI, it was demonstrated that marked protein catabolism was evident following injury for both groups. However, those with TBI did not exhibit worse nitrogen balances than those without TBI. This is in contrast to older studies and may be reflective of improvements in the therapeutic management of patients with TBI, which include the use of propofol and avoidance of corticosteroids. Propofol significantly decreases energy expenditure and may down-regulate the hyper-metabolic-hyper-catabolic response and reduce urinary nitrogen excretion. High-dose corticosteroid therapy, now considered obsolete for the management of TBI, was employed in some earlier studies. Corticosteroids increase nitrogen excretion by as much as 30% to 50%, which may have contributed to the observed exaggerated protein catabolism for TBI patients compared with other groups of trauma patients.

During the acute phase of injury, a nitrogen balance of about –5 g/day or better is sometimes achievable and considered to be near nitrogen equilibrium. Additionally, we measure creatinine clearance during the nitrogen balance determination. The measured creatinine clearance is then compared to predicted creatinine clearance based on the Cockcroft–Gault equations (Table 12.2). For the hyperdynamic, critically ill patient without acute kidney injury or chronic kidney disease, measured creatinine clearance should be at least ~90% or greater than predicted.

Table 12.2 How to calculate and use nitrogen balance

From the case scenario given in Table 1, the patient is prescribed a 1 kcal/mL, 62 g/L protein polymeric enteral formula at 105 mL/hr plus 30 g of protein liquid once daily to achieve a caloric intake of 31 kcal/kg/d and 2.2 g/kg/d of protein. A nitrogen balance is conducted on his fifth day following admission to the trauma ICU. His serum creatinine concentration during the nitrogen balance determination was 0.9 mg/dL and there was no significant change in serum urea nitrogen concentration (from 22 mg/dL to 23 mg/dL). His medication administration record and nursing intake and output record revealed that he received all of his enteral formula (2640 mL or 2.64 L) plus the protein dose during the nitrogen balance. His recorded urine output from the nursing records was similar to that recorded by the laboratory at 2200 mL (2.2 L/d). His urine urea nitrogen concentration was 1300 mg/dL (13 000 mg/L or 13 g/L) and urinary creatinine concentration was 90 mg/dL (900 mg/L). Is this a good goal protein intake for this patient?

Step 1. Check to be sure it was a reasonably accurate collection

Part A. Calculate his predicted creatinine clearance (Cockcroft–Gault equations)

$$pCrCl \ (mL/min) = \frac{(140 - Age) \times Weight \ (kg)}{Serum \ creatinine \ (mg/dL) \times 72} \ (multiply \ results \ by \ 0.85 \ if \ female)$$

$$pCrCl \ (mL/min) = \frac{(140 - 40) \times 85}{0.9 \times 72} = \frac{8500}{64.8} = 131 \ mL/min$$

Part B. Calculate measured creatinine clearance

$$mCrCr \ (mL/min) = \frac{mg \ creatinine/day \times 100}{Serum \ creatinine \times 1440 \ min/day} = \frac{900 \times 2.2 \times 100}{0.9 \times 1440}$$

$$= \frac{198000}{1296} = 153 \ mL/min$$

Part C. Interpretation: Since mCrCL was greater than pCrCL and nursing urine output was close to measured urine output collected, this sample was probably a good collection.

Step 2. Calculate Nitrogen Balance

Part A. Calculate Nitrogen Intake

$$Protein \ intake = (62 \ g/L \ of \ EN \times 2.52 \ L) + 30 \ g \ protein \ (individual \ dose)$$
$$= 156 + 30 = 186 \ g$$

$$Nitrogen \ intake = \frac{Protein \ intake}{6.25*} = \frac{186}{6.25} = 29.8g$$

Part B. Calculate Nitrogen Out

$$Nitrogen \ Out = \frac{Urinary \ Urea \ Nitrogen \ (g/d)}{0.85^\P} + 2 + Body \ Urea$$
$$+ other \ losses \ (drains, \ etc.)$$

$$Nitrogen \ Out = \frac{(13 \times 2.2)}{0.85^\P} + 2 + 0 + 0 = \frac{28.6}{0.85^\P} = 33.6 + 2 = 35.8g$$

Table 12.2 (cont.)

Part C. Calculate Nitrogen Balance

$$\text{Nitrogen Balance} = \text{Nin} - \text{Nout} = 29.8 - 35.8 = -6 \text{ g/d}$$

Step 3. Interpret Nitrogen Balance

This nitrogen balance is probably reasonable for a patient with TBI during the acute phase of the injury especially since he is receiving a protein intake of 2.2 g/kg/d. Some clinicians may increase his protein intake further to ~2.5 g/kg/d to ascertain if nitrogen balance can be further improved since his serum urea nitrogen concentration in the low 20s likely reflects minimal ureagenesis on this protein intake. Other clinicians might be satisfied with this nitrogen balance given his acute phase of injury, current nitrogen balance near nitrogen equilibrium, and given what some clinicians might consider an aggressive protein intake. Whatever option is chosen, it would be reasonable to reassess with another nitrogen balance within the next week to ascertain if a different plan is required for this patient.

*assumes good quality protein (16% nitrogen)

¶ assumes 15% of non-urea nitrogen in urine instead of 2 g which is then added to 2 g stool and integumentary losses per classic nitrogen balance equation: NB = Nin – (UUN + 4) 2 g underestimates non-urea nitrogen in urine for critically ill patients with high urinary nitrogen excretion rates

Body Urea retained calculation accounts for urea retained in the body and is only necessary if a significant SUN change of ~ 4 to 5 mg/dL occurs during the NB determination. Body Urea (g/d) can be estimated by:

$$[(SUN_2 - SUN_1) \times 0.01] \times [\text{Weight (kg)} \times (0.6 \text{ for males, } 0.55 \text{ for females})]$$

SUN, serum urea nitrogen; UUN, urinary urea nitrogen.

In our study with 249 patients, nitrogen equilibrium was more often achieved at protein intakes of 2 g/kg/day or greater. A slowing of nitrogen accretion occurred at protein intakes within 1.7 g/kg/day to 2.2 g/kg/day. Protein intakes in excess of 2.5 g/kg/day resulted in significant ureagenesis, likely caused by net protein catabolism of excess intake.

It is recommended that patients with TBI receive at least 2 g/kg/day of protein without overfeeding with non-protein calories. Our general approach is to design an aggressive protein supplemented regimen whereby the patient will receive within 2 g/kg/day to 2.5 g/kg/day of protein and then follow-up with a nitrogen balance determination. If the nitrogen balance study indicates a balance of ~ −6 or −7 g/day or worse, we may modestly escalate the protein dose in an effort to try to achieve nitrogen equilibrium (−5 g/day or better). Protein doses beyond 2.5 g/kg/day to 3 g/kg/day are unlikely to be effective in improving nitrogen balance significantly and will more likely result in greater ureagenesis. Additionally, we keep the energy goals the same even during marked negative nitrogen balance. Studies have demonstrated the futility of trying to use calories to improve nitrogen balance in critically ill trauma patients and increasing non-protein energy would only be putting the patient at greater risk for the adverse effects of overfeeding.

One scenario in which protein requirements are reduced for those with TBI is in the event the patient is given pentobarbital for management of an elevated ICP refractory to conventional management. Patients given pentobarbital experience a marked reduction in mean urinary nitrogen excretion and energy expenditure of approximately 40% and 50%, respectively. Our current practice is to be restrictive with caloric intake particularly for those in pentobarbital coma to avoid over-feeding. However, we still empirically give ≥2 g/kg/day of protein since the adverse effects of short-term aggressive protein intake are minimal in the absence of renal or hepatic failure.

Glutamine

Glutamine supplementation has been shown to reduce infectious complications, prevent worsened insulin sensitivity, and decrease mortality among critically ill trauma and burned patients. Although the optimal dose of glutamine is not precisely known, most studies indicate a beneficial effect between 0.3 g/kg/day to 0.5 g/kg/day. For patients with TBI, a risk for worse outcomes with glutamine supplementation has been theorized. Astrocytes and other brain cells have the ability to convert glutamine to glutamate via glutaminase. Glutamate is an agonist for the NMDA (N-methyl-di-aspartate) receptor which is thought to be an important regulator for worsening TBI due to secondary ischemic injury, high intracerebral pressure, and edema. Two small recent studies have examined the influence of supplemental intravenous glutamine at 0.34 g/kg/day upon cerebral glutamate concentrations in patients with TBI. Although plasma glutamine concentrations improved by ~30%, intracerebral glutamate concentrations were unaffected with a zero glutamate balance across the brain. Until further data are available, aggressive dosing of glutamine beyond ~ 0.34 g/kg/day is not recommended for patients with TBI.

Selection of an enteral formula

Our approach to enteral nutritional management of patients with isolated TBI or without significant additional injuries (e.g., ISS <20 or ATI <25) is to use a high-protein (e.g., 62 g/L), 1 kcal/mL polymeric formula with additional bolus protein supplementation if necessary (see Table 12.2). Enteral nutrition is usually initiated within 24 to 72 hours of admission to the trauma intensive care unit. For patients with extensive traumatic injuries including TBI, we employ the use of a glutamine-containing, polymeric enteral formula for the first 10 days of nutrition therapy based on our published data indicating decreased infectious complications with the use of a specialized glutamine/arginine/w-3 fatty acid-enriched formula when given to patients with multiple traumatic injuries. Thereafter, we will switch the patient to a high-protein polymeric formulation if continued enteral feeding is required. We generally start EN at about a third of the goal rate and advance by an additional third of the goal rate until the goal is achieved by the third day. Exceptions to this approach may include those with gastric feeding intolerance whereby prokinetic therapy is necessary, severe electrolyte derangements, or those with substantial hyperglycemia whereby a slower escalation in feeding rate combined with aggressive insulin therapy may be preferred.

Glycemic control

Trauma patients have been shown to exhibit improved clinical outcomes from maintaining blood glucose concentrations less than 7.8–8.3 mmol/L, which is tighter than that recommended for other types of critically ill patients. The brain is the most avid glucose consumer of all body organs and severe hypoglycemia (blood glucose <2.2 mmol/L) can produce or exacerbate neurological deficits, encephalopathy, seizures, permanent cognitive dysfunction, and potentially, death. Therefore, extreme caution must be undertaken to avoid hypoglycemia for patients with TBI, and intensive insulin therapy targeting a blood glucose (BG) of 4.5 mmol/L to 6.1 mmol/L is not recommended.

For the hyperglycemic patient with TBI who receives enteral or parenteral nutrition therapy, it is recommended that the exogenous sources of glucose be eliminated if possible. For those receiving enteral nutrition, we employ the use of a "diabetic formula" containing lower amounts of carbohydrate as complex carbohydrates, fiber, and higher lipid content if the glutamine-containing formula is not indicated. We also use intermittent sliding scale regular human insulin coverage every 3 to 4 hours if a continuous infusion is not indicated. If these measures are inadequate for effective glycemic control, then we will employ our paper-based, nurse-driven algorithm (Table 12.3).

Table 12.3 depicts our current and recommended intensive insulin therapy algorithm for glycemic control for patients with traumatic injuries including TBI. We demonstrated that this algorithm could achieve our target BG range of 3.9 to 8.3 mmol/L within 5 hours of initiation and maintain BG concentrations within that range for an average of 20 hours per day. Blood glucose concentrations are monitored every 1 hour with extension to every 2 hours if the patient demonstrates stability in glycemic control and insulin infusion rate. The algorithm should not be used for patients with renal or hepatic failure or others at high risk for hypoglycemia. Additionally, it should not be used for patients who are not receiving continuous intravenous dextrose or enteral carbohydrate. Thus, if the parenteral or enteral nutrition is discontinued for any reason, an intravenous source of dextrose must be given to prevent hypoglycemia.

Fluid and electrolyte considerations

Post-pituitary dysfunction is more prevalent in those with severe TBI than in those with mild or moderate TBI. Resultant aberrations in fluid and sodium homeostasis

Table 12.3 Regular human insulin continuous infusion algorithm*

Blood glucose concentration (mmol/L)	Instructions
<2.2	Stop insulin infusion, give 1 amp D50W, and restart insulin infusion when blood glucose > 5.6 mmol/L at ½ last rate, call MD
2.2–3.9	Stop insulin infusion, give ½ amp D50W, and restart insulin infusion when blood glucose > 5.6 mmol/l at ½ last rate
4.0–5.6	Decrease infusion rate by 50% (round to nearest whole number)
5.7–7.0	No change
7.1–9.8	Increase infusion by 1 unit/hr
9.9–11.2	Increase infusion by 2 units/hr
11.3–12.6	Increase infusion by 3 units/hr
12.7–14.0	Increase infusion by 4 units/hr
14.1–15.4	Increase infusion by 5 units/hr
15.5–16.8	Increase infusion by 6 units/hr
> 16.8	Increase infusion by 6 units/hr and call MD

*Adapted from Dickerson RN, Swiggart CE, Morgan LM, et al. Safety and efficacy of a graduated intravenous insulin infusion protocol in critically ill trauma patients receiving specialized nutritional support. Nutrition 2008;24:536–545.

may contribute to the early morbidity observed for these patients. The most common fluid and sodium perturbations encountered include syndrome of inappropriate anti-diuretic hormone (SIADH), cerebral salt wasting syndrome (CSWS), and diabetes insipidus (DI). Varying levels of chronic post-pituitary dysfunction, particularly SIADH, may occur for a prolonged period for some patients with TBI.

Post-traumatic SIADH or CSWS can result in significant hyponatremia. It is absolutely essential that the clinician identifies the correct pathogenesis for the hyponatremia for the patient with TBI as the treatment of SIADH and CSWS is entirely different. Inappropriate diagnosis could lead to mismanagement of the patient and cause harm. The first step is to exclude other causes of hyponatremia including factitious (or "pseudo") hyponatremia from hyperglycemia or aggressive mannitol intake. The patient must be closely evaluated for excess hypotonic fluid intake, renal or hepatic dysfunction, congestive heart failure, diuretic use, and extracellular fluid volume status.

Hyponatremia, due to SIADH (2% to 37% of patients with TBI), may be due to uncontrolled release of anti-diuretic hormone (also known as arginine vasopressin or AVP) as a result of damage to the pituitary stalk or posterior pituitary gland. It is important to note that there are multiple causes of SIADH during critical illness in addition to TBI including pain, medications, stress, pneumonia, infections, certain malignancies, hypothyroidism, and adrenal insufficiency that must also be ruled out in the differential diagnosis. SIADH may be confused with CSWS. Although

Table 12.4 Clinical findings in syndrome of inappropriate anti-diuretic hormone (SIADH) versus cerebral salt wasting syndrome (CSWS)*

SIADH	SCWS
Hyponatremia	Hyponatremia
Normal or slightly expanded ECF volume	Decreased ECF volume
Sodium equilibrium (may be variable)	Negative sodium balance
Positive fluid balance or fluid equilibrium	Negative fluid balance
Serum osmolality decreased	Serum osmolality increased
Urine osmolality increased	Urine osmolality increased
Urine sodium increased (>40 mmol/L)	Urine sodium markedly increased (>80 mmol/L)
Increased weight	Decreased weight

ECF, extracellular fluid.
* Adapted from: Dickerson RN. Hyponatremia in neurosurgical patients: syndrome of inappropriate antidiuretic hormone or cerebral salt wasting syndrome? Hospital Pharmacy 2002;37:1336–1341.

there are exceptions, the development of SIADH usually occurs within the first week to 10 days for TBI patients and CSWS usually occurs approximately in the second week following injury. Table 12.4 summarizes the clinical findings associated with SIADH and CSWS.

The appropriate management for the hyponatremic patient with SIADH is fluid restriction, including a reduction in intravenous fluids, oral fluids, and concentration of the parenteral or enteral nutrition regimen. To restrict fluid intake with parenteral nutrition, solutions should be compounded using 70% dextrose, 15% or 20% amino acids, 20% to 30% lipid emulsion solutions and to limit the addition of free water to the PN solution. For enteral nutrition, a concentrated (2 kcal/mL) enteral formula may be required. If fluid restriction is unsuccessful, sodium chloride may be added to the enteral or parenteral nutrition to make its final sodium concentration near 140 mmol/L to 150 mmol/L. For the patient refractory to conventional management, use of an arginine vasopressin antagonist such as conivaptan or tolvaptan can also be initiated. A single 20 mg intravenous bolus dose of conivaptan can increase serum sodium concentration by 4 mmol/L in a 24-hour period. This technique may be safer for hyponatremic patients than conventional dosing of conivaptan (e.g., bolus dose followed by a 4-day continuous infusion) as rises in serum sodium concentration are not likely to exceed 12 mmol/L per day with the manufacturer-recommended infusion method. This is important as a rapid rise in serum sodium concentration (>12 mmol/L/day) can lead to central pontine myelinolysis and death.

For the patient with CSWS, addition of sodium to the parenteral nutrition solution or to the enteral formulation is required. We empirically add up to 150 mmol/L of sodium (as chloride, acetate, or a mixture of sodium chloride with acetate including phosphate depending on the acid–base status of the patient) to the parenteral nutrition solution. For patients receiving enteral nutrition formulas, we will add ~ 100 mmol/L of sodium chloride to the enteral feeding formula (to achieve a total of ~ 150 mmol/L of Na in the enteral feeding solution) or give the patient sodium chloride tablets per the feeding tube.

Central DI associated with TBI results in a lack of production of AVP due to damage to the hypothalamus or post-pituitary gland. It occurs in about 3% of patients with severe TBI. The diagnosis of DI following TBI in the post-operative period may be difficult because polyuria can occur during this period secondary to a variety of causes including mannitol, hyperglycemia, ureagenesis, or mobilization of excessive resuscitation fluid. If the DI is not identified and treated early, severe dehydration and life-threatening hypernatremia can rapidly ensue. Central DI may occur within a few days after injury and is detected by a voluminous urine output of >300 mL/hour with hypotonic urine (urine specific gravity <1.05 or urine osmolality <150 mOsm/kg). Treatment of central DI requires the supplementation of exogenous AVP, namely DDAVP (desmopressin acetate) 1–2 μg subcutaneously or intravenously twice daily or vasopressin 10 units subcutaneously twice (up to four times) daily depending on patient response according to urine output. Slow replacement of lost fluid is recommended with close monitoring of serum sodium concentration (e.g., every 6 hours). The serum sodium concentration should not fall more than 10–12 mmol/L in a day and preferably slower to prevent worsening of cerebral edema. Provision of intravenous hypotonic ¼ normal saline (0.225% sodium chloride) solution is discouraged as recent data suggests evidence of minor hemolysis even with central venous administration. Intravenous D5 ¼ NS or ½ NS or D5W and/or intra-gastric water boluses (if tolerated) would be a more preferable replacement fluid solution under most circumstances.

Intracellular electrolyte requirements, especially phosphorus, potassium, and magnesium, are markedly increased for patients with TBI compared to other critically ill patients. Studies have reported that patients with severe TBI have a higher incidence of hypophosphatemia <0.65 mmol/L (e.g., 61% versus 0%), hypokalemia <3.6 mmol/L (e.g., 44% versus 5%), and hypomagnesemia <0.62 mmol/L (e.g., 67% versus 11%) when compared to other trauma patients. It is our practice to commonly provide supplemental phosphorus, potassium, and sometimes magnesium or calcium therapy to these patients. Table 12.5 depicts our conventional intravenous intracellular electrolyte dosing requirements for trauma patients. Of particular note is the differentiation between phosphorus dosing for patients with TBI in contrast to other critically ill patients. In addition to aggressive supplemental intravenous phosphorus doses, we will often add 30 mmol of either sodium or potassium phosphate per liter of enteral or parenteral feeding.

Table 12.5 Intravenous electrolyte dosing for critically ill patients with traumatic injuries including TBI (these doses should NOT be used for patients with renal impairment)

A. Phosphorus

Serum phosphorus concentration (mmol/L)	Dosage (mmol/kg) for TBI, trauma, and burn patients	Dosage (mmol/kg) for other patients
0.74–0.97	0.32	0.16
0.49–0.73	0.64	0.32
<0.49	1	0.64

The drug should be mixed in 100 to 250 ml of 0.9% sodium chloride or D5W and given at a rate no faster than 7.5 mmol/hr. Potassium phosphate salt can be used for patients with a serum potassium <4.0 (3 mmol P = 4.4 mmol K). Sodium phosphate salt should be used for patients with a serum potassium ≥4.0 (3 mmol P = 4 mmol Na). Increase phosphate content of EN/PN if possible.

B. Potassium

For an "average" size (e.g., 65–90 kg) patient with normal renal function and without excessive losses (e.g., furosemide, amphotericin B, etc.). These doses should NOT be used for patients with renal impairment or adrenal insufficiency. Serum magnesium concentrations should be assessed in any hypokalemic patient. Increase potassium content of EN/PN/IV fluids if possible.

Serum K (mmol/L)	KCl dosage (mmol/L)
3.5–3.9	40 mmol × 1 dose
3.0–3.4	40 mmol × 2 doses
2.0–2.9	40 mmol × 3 doses

IV KCl doses should be given only by central vein. KCl can be given at 20 mmol/hr if patient has continuous ECG monitoring in the ICU. 10 mmol/hr is safest if patient is asymptomatic or not in the ICU. Peripheral intravenous solutions should not contain more than 40 to 60 mmol of KCl/L. Alteration of the above doses may be necessary depending on the patient's body size.

C. Magnesium

Serum Mg (mmol/L)	Dose (g/kg)
0.66–0.74	0.05
0.41–0.65	0.1
<0.41	0.15

The drug should be mixed in 100 to 250 mL of normal saline or D5W and given at a rate no faster than 1 g (4 mmol) per hour. Successful treatment of hypomagnesemia usually takes 3 to 5 days of therapy. Magnesium concentrations are often elevated for 1–2 days following an infusion because it takes about 48 hours for the magnesium to fully redistribute to the body tissues.

Table 12.5 (cont.)

D. Calcium

Calcium may be falsely low in the presence of hypoalbuminemia. For every 1 g/dL fall in serum albumin below 4.0, serum calcium will fall by about 0.2 mmol/L. With low serum albumin concentrations and during critical illness, this relationship may not be precise and obtaining an ionized calcium level is recommended. Serum magnesium concentrations should be assessed in any hypocalcemic patient.

Ionized calcium (mmol/L)	Calcium dosage (g)
1.00–1.12	2 g calcium gluconate over 2 hours
≤0.99	4 g calcium gluconate over 4 hours

The drug should be mixed in 100 mL NSS or D5W over 1–2 hours; increase in PN solution. Can be given as a slow i.v. push if necessary; infusion is safer. Increase in PN solution if possible.

Drug–nutrient interactions (phenytoin)

The most common potential drug–nutrient interaction among critically ill patients with TBI who receive enteral feeding is with phenytoin. Phenytoin is routinely given for the first week following severe TBI for seizure prophylaxis. To avoid decreases in serum phenytoin concentrations when co-administered with continuous intra-gastric feeding or to prevent discontinuation of feeding prior to phenytoin administration, we opt to continue intravenous administration of phenytoin throughout the 7-day prophylaxis period.

Spinal cord injury

The major causes for traumatic SCI are motor vehicle collisions and falls which account for over two-thirds of all cases each year. The metabolic management of the critically ill patient with SCI can be challenging due to sequelae from the injury as well as other associated complications common in this patient population including denervation atrophy and paralysis, glucose intolerance, neurogenic shock, pneumonia, skin breakdown, neurogenic bowel and bladder, gastric ulcerations, venous thromboembolism, and bone hyper-resorption. During the acute phase post-injury while the patient requires mechanical ventilation, enteral nutrition or parenteral nutrition (if the patient cannot be fed enterally) is required. Although only data from small trials are available, no major complications have been reported with early enteral feeding commenced within 2 to 3 days post-injury. Since patients with SCI often have other traumatic injuries, it is our practice to provide early metabolic support and by the enteral route whenever possible.

Energy requirements

Patients with SCI tend to be hypometabolic with resting energy expenditures less than predicted by, e.g., the Harris–Benedict equation. Patients have a reduced energy expenditure due to lowered sympathetic nervous system activity (determined by measurement of energy expenditure and adjusting for fat-free mass and age) as well as reduced levels of physical activity. Patients with SCI also have been shown to have a slightly reduced thermogenic response to food intake (e.g., specific dynamic action) from 15% to about 12% when compared to controls. Analogous to the adult patient with cerebral palsy, SCI patients with quadriplegia are more hypometabolic than those with paraplegia (with maintenance of upper body mobility and movement). Cox (1985) found measured resting energy expenditure of stable, rehabilitating patients with SCI to be 23 kcal/kg/day if they were quadriplegic and 28 kcal/kg/day if paraplegic. Recent literature emphasizing obesity interventions in persons with SCI mandates a conservative approach with caloric dosing to avoid complications from overfeeding of gaining excessive weight (e.g., decubitus ulcer formation) or obesity (e.g., diabetes, cardiovascular disease). Empirically a caloric intake of 80% to 100% of predicted (Harris–Benedict equations) should be provided for those with quadriplegia and 100% to 120% for those with paraplegia. Patients should be closely monitored for evidence of overfeeding and serial weight measurements. An assessment of change in total body fat, by anthropometry or bioelectrical impedance, might also be helpful in assessing adequacy of the caloric intake during the rehabilitation phase of their therapy.

Protein requirements

Patients with SCI often display massive urinary nitrogen losses and yet remain unresponsive to nutrition therapy due to immobility and denervation muscle atrophy. It is not uncommon in our practice to observe a multiple trauma patient with quadriplegia who experiences a nitrogen balance of −10 g/day or worse despite receiving ≥2 g/kg/day of protein intake while in the ICU. Other studies have confirmed these findings and it is therefore accepted that a negative nitrogen balance is obligatory for these patients and attempting to achieve a positive nitrogen balance by grossly escalating protein and energy intake may result in overfeeding complications. Although it is unknown how much protein is required to help them recover from their other injuries, heal wounds, and support a functioning immunological response to infections, we empirically provide about 2 g/kg/day of protein based on the anticipated needs of other trauma patients.

Glycemic control

In addition to insulin resistance and increased gluconeogenesis from traumatic stress or infection, patients with SCI are sometimes given intravenous glucocorticoids for the first 24 to 48 hours following admission to the ICU. This practice is not recommended by the AANS/CNS Joint Section on Disorders of the Spine and

Peripheral Nerves guidelines. According to the National Acute Spinal Cord Injury Study (NACIS) group corticosteroids failed to demonstrate clinical benefits in non-penetrating SCI and may be potentially harmful to the patient (increased infections). From the metabolic support standpoint, addition of aggressive short-term glucocorticoid (methylprednisolone) therapy may result in loss of glycemic control. To manage hyperglycemia for these patients, we use a low carbohydrate, high-fat enteral or parenteral regimen, omit dextrose from other intravenous sources, and provide intravenous regular human insulin sliding scale coverage every 3 to 4 hours. If these techniques are unsuccessful and the hyperglycemia is severe and/or prolonged, then we will consider the use of intensive insulin therapy as outlined in Table 12.3.

Neurogenic shock and enteral nutrition

The incidence of neurogenic shock (hypotension, bradycardia, decreased vascular resistance) for isolated SCI is approximately 19% in cervical cord injuries and 7% and 3% in thoracic and lumbar cord injuries, respectively. An adequate blood pressure is thought to maintain adequate perfusion to the injured spinal cord and limit secondary ischemic injury. Thus, intravenous fluids and vasopressor therapy are given to maintain adequate blood pressure during neurogenic shock. Controversy exists whether patients should be fed enterally when receiving significant vasopressor therapy. The theoretical concern is that with high doses of vasopressors, blood flow will be shunted from the mesenteric vascular beds predisposing the patient to intestinal ischemia if enteral feeding is attempted. Enteral feeding is thought to require additional energy and increased blood flow and perfusion to the gastrointestinal tract for peristalsis and absorption of nutrients. Case reports of necrotic bowel from small bowel enteral feeding in patients with hemodynamic instability have been reported. Unfortunately, there is a paucity of literature regarding enteral feeding tolerance, intestinal ischemia, and vasopressor use for patients with SCI. Given the theoretical concerns and the lack of data, the safety of early enteral feeding for patients with SCI and neurogenic shock remains an enigma. Our empirical approach has been to attempt intra-gastric feeding for the SCI patient with neurogenic shock whose blood pressure and heart rate is effectively maintained by the use of dopamine and/or norepinephrine. If the patient demonstrates intolerance to the feeding (e.g., high gastric residual volumes, abdominal distension) or if the patient's blood pressure is extremely labile requiring large and/or variable doses of vasopressors, we will consider implementation of parenteral nutrition. It is recommended that conventional practice should consist of a conservative approach to enteral feeding during neurogenic shock until more definitive studies are published.

Neurogenic bowel

Neurogenic bowel dysfunction may result in incontinence or constipation or fecal retention depending on whether the patient experiences lower (areflexive) or upper (hyperreflexive) motor bowel dysfunction. Bowel training usually consists of docusate (a stool softener), a colonic stimulant that stimulates Auerbach's plexus to induce peristalsis (e.g., senna), and a contact irritant in the mucosa of the colon (e.g., bisacodyl). A typical bowel training program is docusate 100 mg twice to three times daily, senna 15 mg one or two tablets daily, and bisacodyl 10 mg per rectum or per tube daily. Sometimes, an enema is required if the patient does not have a bowel movement within a couple of days. Long-term use of stimulant laxatives such as senna and cascara are avoided by some clinicians in an effort to avoid potential neuropathic damage to the myenteric plexus. Alternative osmotic agents such as lactulose or polyethylene glycol may be preferred for long-term use. A regular schedule of bowel movements is important as the absence of stools can result in rendering the colon less plastic, causing distension and reducing the effectiveness of peristalsis. Some patients will require adjustments in their medications depending on the frequency and consistency of the stool. It is recommended that a fiber-containing enteral formula (at least 30 g of dietary fiber/day) be selected for long-term use in the patient with SCI who is unable to be fed orally. For patients with fecal incontinence and diarrhea, additional fiber supplementation including psyllium may be required.

Bone hyper-resorption

Metabolic bone disease is associated with the chronic critically ill patient including those with TBI, SCI, and thermal injury. This is particularly pertinent for those who are bedridden and immobile without adequate sunlight exposure. Patients usually present with hyperphosphatemia, increased urinary N-telopeptide (collagen breakdown product from bone) and increased calciuria, suppressed parathyroid hormone and 1,25-dihydroxyvitamin D concentrations, and occasionally with intermittent hypercalcemia. Heterotopic ossification occurs in 16% to 53% of patients with SCI and evidence of significant bone resorption has been reported as early as 9 days post SCI. Treatment includes concurrent pamidronate 30 mg i.v. daily for 3 days, 0.25 to 0.5 μg calcitriol orally/per tube daily, and 1000 mg of elemental calcium orally/per tube daily. Additional calcium supplementation beyond 1000 mg daily and phosphorus supplementation is often indicated as post-bisphosphonate (pamidronate or etidronate) hypocalcemia and hypophosphatemia has been reported to occur in 44% and 53% of SCI patients, respectively. Oral etidronate (20 mg/kg), calcitriol, and calcium therapy is often continued for 6 months following SCI by some clinicians.

Summary points

- Gastric feeding intolerance in patients with traumatic brain injury is twice that of other trauma patients.
- Total energy requirements are increased in patients with traumatic brain injury. Protein should be administered at 2–2.5 g/kg/day and nitrogen balance monitored.

- Combination therapy of metoclopramide and erythromycin reduces tachyphylaxis of prokinetic monotherapy.
- Medications used for therapy and sedation may affect energy requirements in patients with traumatic brain injury.
- Patients with SCI are hypometabolic and will exhibit negative nitrogen balance.

Further reading

Bratton SL, Chestnut RM, Ghajar J, et al. Guidelines for the management of severe traumatic brain injury. XII. Nutrition. J Neurotrauma 2007;24 (Suppl 1):S77–82.

Cook AM, Peppard A, Magnuson B. Nutrition considerations in traumatic brain injury. Nutr Clin Pract 2008;23:608–620.

Cox SA, Weiss SM, Posuniak EA, et al. Energy expenditure after spinal cord injury: an evaluation of stable rehabilitating patients. J Trauma 1985;25(5):419–423.

Dickerson RN. Hyponatremia in neurosurgical patients: syndrome of inappropriate antidiuretic hormone or cerebral salt wasting syndrome? Hospital Pharmacy 2002;37:1336–1341.

Dickerson RN, Swiggart CE, Morgan LM, et al. Safety and efficacy of a graduated intravenous insulin infusion protocol in critically ill trauma patients receiving specialized nutritional support. Nutrition 2008;24:536–545.

Dickerson RN, Mitchell JN, Morgan LM, et al. Disparate response to metoclopramide therapy for gastric feeding intolerance in trauma patients with and without traumatic brain injury. J Parenter Enteral Nutr 2009;33:646–655.

Dickerson RN, Pitts SL, Maish GO, 3rd, et al. A reappraisal of nitrogen requirements for patients with critical illness and trauma. J Trauma 2012;73:549–557.

Hadley MN. Nutritional support after spinal cord injury. Neurosurgery 2002;50(Suppl 3): S81–84.

Lindsey KA, Brown RO, Maish GO 3rd, Croce MA, Minard G, Dickerson RN. Influence of traumatic brain injury on potassium and phosphorus homeostasis in critically ill multiple trauma patients. Nutrition 2010;26:784–790.

Ruf K, Magnuson B, Hatton J, Cook AM. Nutrition in neurologic impairment. In: Mueller CM (ed) The A.S.P.E.N. Adult Nutrition Support Core Curriculum, 2nd ed. Silver Spring: American Society for Parenteral and Enteral Nutrition; 2012: 363–376.

Stiens SA, Bergman SB, Goetz LL. Neurogenic bowel dysfunction after spinal cord injury: clinical evaluation and rehabilitative management. Arch Phys Med Rehabil 1997;78 (3 Suppl):S86–102.

13

Nutritional support of critically ill immuno-compromised patients

Peter K. Linden

Introduction

In the last several decades, patients with critical illness who are immuno-compromised due either to native diseases and/or iatrogenic immuno-suppression comprise a rising proportion of the patient census in both surgical and medical intensive care units. Major disease categories include those with solid – or hematogenous cancers receiving chemotherapy, radiation and/or surgical intervention, solid – and liquid (bone marrow) – organ recipients, acquired immunodeficiency syndrome, burn patients, and patients on longstanding immuno-suppression for autoimmune disease. The prevention, diagnosis, and management of opportunistic infection in such patients has always been of paramount concern for critical care clinicians to preserve a favorable patient outcome. However, the appropriate timing, delivery route, and quantity and quality of nutritional support are clearly critical but difficult elements of care since there are patients who also exhibit multiple obstacles to these goals (Table 13.1).

In the critically ill, the paradigm for nutritional support has been transformed from a supportive, replacement one to an active modulatory strategy. The majority of such investigation has focused on counteracting the severe catabolism during the pro-inflammatory, acute phase response and subsequently modulating the acquired state of immuno-suppression due to immuno-paralysis and counter-inflammatory, down-regulation in patients with critical illness due to trauma, severe infection and sepsis, major surgery, and other severe stress states. Despite the proliferation of immuno-modulatory feeding formulas there have been very few randomized trials of nutritional support in homogeneous populations of patients with the orthodox immuno-compromised states discussed herein. Indeed although the evidence database from the 2009 SCCM-ASPEN and 2003 Canadian clinical practice guidelines for nutritional support in critical illness did include some randomized trials in immuno-compromised hosts (principally surgical oncology patients and burn patients) their recommendations were all based upon a heterogeneous mix of mostly

Nutrition in Critical Care, ed. Peter Faber and Mario Siervo. Published by Cambridge University Press. © Cambridge University Press 2014.

Table 13.1 Challenges and obstacles to achieving adequate nutrition in the critically ill immuno-compromised patient

---

Poor specificity of nutritional status assessments
Anthropometric measurements
Pre-existing lymphocyte depletion
Anergy skin testing
Circulating proteins (albumin, pre-albumin, transferrin)

Delivery access for nutrition
Nasal-enteral access tubes associated with sinusitis, hemorrhage with blood dyscrasia
Enhanced risk for infection in vascular access sites
Gastroparesis in diabetic patients, upper GI surgery, and abdominal organ recipients
Chemotherapy-induced nausea/vomiting
High risk for percutaneous gastrostomy

Alimentary tract dysfunction
Oral and intestinal mucositis following chemotherapy
Compromised gut function (small bowel transplant, HIV enteropathy)
Graft-versus-host disease involving intestines
Post-transplant allograft organ dysfunction – kidney, liver, lung
Mechanical bowel obstruction

Metabolic considerations
High prevalence of pre-existing catabolism and cachexia (HIV, cancer)
Corticosteroid-related glucose intolerance
Pre-existing malnourishment due to anorexia, dysphagia
Trace element deficiency
Poor hepatic function (liver recipients, cardiomyopathy, solid tumor)

Impaired immune response
Sensitivity to exogenous organisms (water, probiotics)
Role of immune-enhancing formula in organ recipients (?)
Infection risk with probiotics

Drug–nutrition interaction
Immuno-suppression-induced diarrhea (mycophenolate)
Reduced bioavailability – HAART, ciclosporin, tacrolimus

---

immuno-competent and a smaller number of immuno-compromised but critically ill patients. With only limited high level evidence derived purely from the study of orthodox immuno-compromised hosts one must extrapolate which nutritional support and modulation strategies are rational, efficacious, and safe in these special patient categories. Thus clinicians who care for critically ill patients with major immuno-compromise in systemic host defenses should pose the question, "what is the general applicability of the major society guidelines for solid- and liquid organ recipients, chemotherapy-treated cancer patients, and AIDS patients?" Intuitively, the major goals of nutrition support in critically ill orthodox immuno-compromised hosts are no different than for immuno-competent patients but there may exist a higher degree of difficulty in these special patients (Table 13.2). These include early

Table 13.2 Major goals in the nutritional support of the critically ill immuno-compromised patient

Restore–maintain lean body mass
Calorie provision commensurate with ideal weight and stressed energy expenditure
Titrate nutrition composition to co-existing organ failure(s)
Maintain gut integrity
Trace mineral replacement of deficits and ongoing losses
Use delivery methods which minimize risks of infection, bleeding
Immune-enhancement formulas when appropriate
Glucose control
Guarantee adequate delivery of enteral ancillary medications
– anti-retrovirals
– immunosuppressive agents
– anti-infectious agents
Prevent exposure to hospital-acquired pathogens during delivery

enteral support, limiting parenteral support to cases where enteral support is not safely achievable, provision of caloric and protein goals, micronutrient repletion, and utilization of immune-enhancing formulas (omega 3 fatty acids, arginine, glutamine, nucleotide, and antioxidants) in appropriate patients.

Pre-existing nutritional deficiency in immuncompromised hosts

Nutritional deficiency states are ubiquitous amongst immuno-compromised patients even prior to medical or surgical conditions, which results in critical illness. Cancer patients are frequently malnourished due to anorexia, the mechanical-obstructive effects of head and neck and gastrointestinal tumors, and advanced lean muscle mass wasting due to catabolic cytokine effects (interleukins-1 and -6, tumor necrosis factor). Prior to solid organ transplantation many prospective recipients have protein energy malnutrition with loss of both lean muscle mass and subcutaneous fat. End stage liver disease patients have a prevalence of protein–energy malnutrition from 20% to 100% with more severe malnourishment in patients with advanced cirrhosis, ascites, porto-systemic encephalopathy, and alcohol-related liver disease. Severe pre-transplant malnutrition status of the liver recipient has been associated with inferior patient and graft survival. HIV-1-related disease is commonly associated with both starvation and cachexia. Manifestations include lean muscle wastage, lipodystrophy, intestinal enteropathy with secondary malabsorption of both macro- and micronutrients (vitamin A, B6, B12 and D, iron, zinc, selenium), and a 10–20% increase in REE due to chronic pro-inflammatory cytokine aberrations. Partial immune restoration with highly active anti-retroviral treatment (HAART) has been shown to modify or reverse muscle wastage, HIV-1-related enteropathy, and catabolism so prevalent in the pre-HAART era.

Conversely, HAART has been shown to be less effective if severe nutritional deficits remain uncorrected and has also been shown to cause lipodystrophy and glucose intolerance. Micronutrient (mineral and vitamin) deficiencies are commonly present or rapidly develop with critical illness due to compromised dietary intake, poor absorption, and increased losses. Although commonly utilized, formal assessments of nutritional status in critically ill immuno-compromised hosts may be misleading due to accumulation of extracellular fluid, which maintains weight and limb circumference, diminished synthesis of hepatic proteins and antibodies, disease- and therapy-related lymphopenia, and increased unmeasured non-urinary nitrogen losses. The SGA scale remains a highly reliable tool as it is a balanced assay of history, physical, and functional data and is not reliant upon spot laboratory values.

Delivery access, timing, and quantity of nutritional support

The reduction in infectious complications associated with early initiation of enteral tube feedings vs either no feedings or parenteral nutrition should be an attractive feature in critically ill immuno-compromised hosts. Although the majority of large randomized trials showing this association were performed in immuno-competent patients (trauma, gastrointestinal surgery, and pancreatitis) similar benefits with early enteral nutrition, including maintenance of gut permeability barrier function, intestinal villous height, gut-associated lymphoid tissue, decreased pro-inflammatory cytokines and reducing metabolic and infectious complications of parenteral nutrition, remain important priorities. However, there are several important aspects to consider when enteral nutrition is started in some specific immuno-compromised hosts. In coagulopathic patients with myelo-suppression or liver disease, placement and maintenance of a nasoenteric feeding tube has an enhanced risk for epistaxis. Even following successful placement of a nasoenteric tube maintaining the access is often difficult in chemotherapy- and radiation-treated patients due to tube dislodgement from severe nausea/vomiting, hemorrhage due to mucositis-related ulceration in the nasopharynx, oropharynx or esophagus, and sinus ostia occlusion resulting in sinus infection in neutropenic patients. Thus when possible, a nasoenteric feeding tube should be placed preemptively, i.e., just prior to myelo-suppressive and emesis-inducing chemotherapy. In cancer patients, recent chemotherapy or radiation therapy commonly exhibit severe upper gastrointestinal intolerance due to pro-emetic side effects of treatment which may be refractory to routine and high-dose anti-emetic, pro-motility agents. However it is often difficult to distinguish whether the failure to tolerate enteral feedings is more the effect of the feeding process or simply refractory chemotherapy-related gastrointestinal intolerance. Percutaneous gastrostomy (PEG) or jejunostomy (PEJ) tubes are a good option in carefully selected cases such as head and neck cancer resections, esophagectomy patients, intestinal transplants, and those with refractory gastroparesis; however the timing of

Table 13.3 Indications for parenteral nutrition in critically ill immuno-compromised hosts

General states
  Refractory ileus
  Severe infectious enteritis
  Bowel perforation, fistulas
  Unrelieved mechanical small bowel obstruction

Solid organ transplant recipients
  Intestinal transplant – until post-transplant anastomotic healing
  Intestinal allograft dysfunction (ischemia, rejection)

Bone marrow recipients
  During engraftment period if enteral attempts unsuccessful
  Severe graft-versus-host disease

Cancer
  Chemotherapy–radiation enteritis refractory to enteral attempts
  Typhlitis

HIV-1 infection
  Refractory HIV enteropathy
  Advanced enteric infections – cryptosporidiosis, mycobacterium

tube placement must be outside the period of severe myelosuppression and heightened bleeding risk. Standard nutrient goals for the critically ill patient (25–30 calories/kg/day, 1.5 g protein/kg/day, fat 30–40% of calories with a balanced long-chain and medium-chain composition, and 60–70% carbohydrate calories) remain broadly applicable to immuno-compromised patients. However higher caloric and protein intakes may be indicated in severe stress, mucositis and other malabsorptive enteropathy, and profound pre-existing lean mass wasting at the onset of critical illness (HIV-1, cirrhosis). Although the clinical bias increasingly supports enteral nutrition as the "default preference" in all immuno-compromised hosts there are a limited number of scenarios where parenteral nutrition remains the only option, which are summarized in Table 13.3. To minimize the adverse sequelae of parenteral nutrition it is paramount that the clinician begins TPN with a prospective plan to correct the factor(s) which necessitated its use.

Specific immuno-compromised host types

Bone marrow transplant recipients

Amongst all immuno-compromised hosts, bone marrow recipients represent the greatest challenge in achieving adequate and safe enteral nutrition. All categories of bone marrow transplantation including allogenic, autologous,

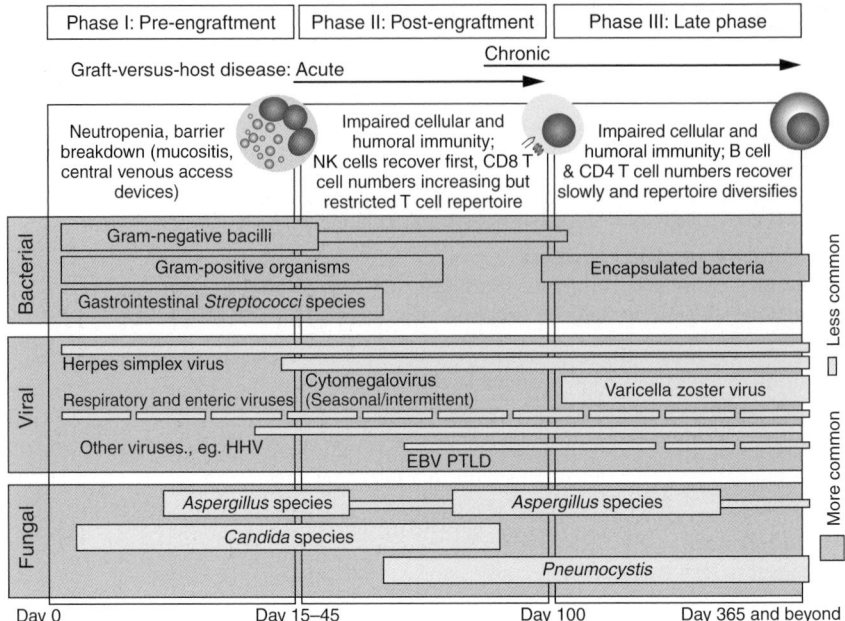

Phase I: Pre-engraftment	Phase II: Post-engraftment	Phase III: Late phase

Figure 13.1 Temporal immune defects and common opportunistic infections following allogenic bone marrow transplantation. (Reproduced from Tomblyn M, Chiller T, Einsele H, et al. Guidelines for preventing infectious complications among hematopoietic cell transplantation recipients: a global perspective. Biology of Blood and Marrow Transplantation 2009;15(10):1143–1238, with permission from Elsevier.)

peripheral blood progenitor (stem) cell, and cord blood transplantation require a pre-transplant ablative chemotherapeutic-radiation conditioning regimen followed by immunosuppressive prophylaxis of graft-versus-host disease (GVHD) with either cyclosporine, corticosteroids, or methotrexate, which results in a protracted period of immuno-suppression and vulnerability to a diverse spectrum of pathogens (Figure 13.1).

The time delay to bone marrow engraftment is the most severe period of immuno-suppression with neutropenia serving as the dominant immune defect (absolute neutrophil count < 500/mm^3). Neutropenia is most prolonged in allogenic and autologous methods where duration to successful engraftment may be as long as 14–21 days while the use of growth factors and peripheral stem cell sources has reduced this period to 7 days. The gastrointestinal tract sustains collateral damage within 7–10 days with oral, esophageal, and intestinal mucositis (Figure 13.2) which may manifest as severe pain, odynophagia, refractory nausea–vomiting, abdominal distension, bleeding, diarrhea, and nutrient malabsorption for a period until bone marrow engraftment (usually 2–3 weeks) or longer with delayed engraftment.

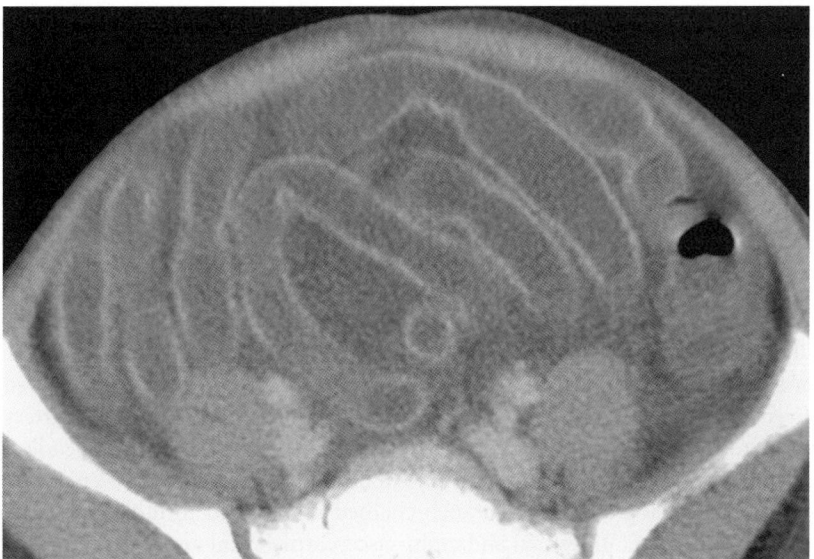

Figure 13.2 Abdominal CT scan of chemotherapy patient with severe intestinal mucositis.

Although it portends successful engraftment, acute GVHD may cause another period of nutritional compromise, occurring within the first 100 days after transplant, and usually involves the small and large intestines, manifesting as a secretory diarrhea, bleeding, and even intestinal perforation. In the critically ill subset of bone marrow recipients who require intensive care admission adequate oral nutrition intake is rarely if ever feasible. Moreover, energy expenditure as high as 130–150% of predicted basal requirements (30–40 kcal/kg/day) has been measured by calorimetry. Despite its well known drawbacks parenteral nutrition has been the traditionally preferred route of nutritional support to bridge the period of severe mucositis, neutropenia, and inter-current critical illness at the majority of bone marrow transplant centers. The ubiquitous presence of a tunneled or non-tunneled central venous access has in part facilitated this practice. In more recent years a pro–con dichotomy of opinion has evolved with regards to the optimal (parenteral vs enteral) route of nutrition in bone marrow recipients. In a meta-analysis including 19 trials of cancer patients including four bone marrow transplant trials, TPN-managed patients had a 16% greater risk of infection, 40% risk of total complications, and lower chemo-therapy response rates. Advocates of enteral nutrition point to the shorter time to gut recovery, reduced bacteremia-bacterial translocation rates, avoidance of the enhanced risk of central line related bacterial and *Candida* infection when hyper-alimentation is being administered via the line, and lower rates of diuretic use, hyperglycemia, and subclavian thromboses. In the absence of high level evidence for the critically ill subset the decision to use enteral or parenteral or combined support still needs to be individualized on a case-by-case basis.

Solid organ transplant recipients

The majority of solid organ recipients enter the post-transplant period with some degree of malnourishment but in the absence of peri-operative complications most can assume a volitional oral diet in the early post-operative period. Liver recipients have biliary reconstruction with either a direct duct-to-duct anastomosis (choledoch-choledochostomy) or the donor duct is implanted into a roux Y limb of recipient jejunum (choledochojejunostomy). Patients with a choledocho-jejunostomy require a 3–5 day delay if gastric feedings are to be employed. Enteral feedings are prudent in severely cachectic patients, those with persistent large volume ascites, and patients with poor allograft function due to technical complications, preservation injury, or severe rejection. Lipid intolerance may be observed in liver recipients who undergo extensive peri-aortic dissection for hepatic artery grafting resulting in lymphatic insufficiency and chylous ascites or severe choles-tasis due to ischemic preservation injury manifesting as diarrhea. Even in the setting of liver allograft failure, branch-chained amino acid formulas have not shown a clear benefit. Intestinal and multi-visceral transplant are virtually unique as almost all such patients are already on long-term parenteral nutrition support at the time of transplantation, which is restarted within 24–48 hours after transplantation for a 7–14 day period when the absorptive capacity of the transplanted intestine recovers. An overlapping period of gastrostomy or jejunostomy tube feedings titrated to avoid excessive ileal stoma output are then begun to allow weaning off the parenteral nutrition. Elemental or peptide-based protein formulas with a medium-chain triglyceride lipid component are usually preferred due to a relative peptidase deficiency and the loss of lymphatic drainage capacity in the intestinal allograft. Despite a high immunosuppressive burden, symptomatic intestinal allograft rejection is very common and may necessitate a temporary return to parenteral nutrition if ileus or high stomal output ensues. Pancreas and pancreas–kidney transplant patients with selectively severe type I diabetes mellitus have a very high incidence of diabetic gastroparesis which may not wane with the achievement of exogenous insulin-free normoglycemia. Although more concentrated enteral formulas are an attractive option with severe gastroparesis, their high lipid content may further delay gastric emptying and can aggravate post-transplant ischemic pancreatitis. Endoscopic or fluoroscopic guided nasoduodenal or nasojejunal feeding tubes are especially valuable options in such cases.

What is the role of immune-modulating formulas?

Meta-analysis data have shown that enteral formulas supplemented with gluta-mine, arginine, nucleic acid, omega-3 fatty acids, and antioxidants reduce infectious complications but not overall mortality in a diverse spectrum of critically ill populations. Immuno-compromised groups which were incorporated into these analyses included burn patients, and head-and neck and gastrointestinal–lung cancer patients undergoing surgery. Extrapolating such results to other non-studied categories of immuno-compromised patients, such as bone marrow transplant and solid organ recipients where iatrogenic immuno-suppression is usually a therapeutic goal, remains difficult. Immune-enhancing formulas are in fact specifically contraindicated in solid organ transplant recipients although evidence that they can independently cause allograft rejection is lacking. Since the studied immune-enhancing formulas all contain multiple components it is difficult to ascribe outcome results to an individual component. Notably, solely administered glutamine has been the most intensively studied in bone marrow transplant and chemotherapy patients. In small studies, dipeptide glutamine-supplemented parenteral feedings have shown beneficial effects on intestinal mucosal integrity and function following radiation therapy and chemotherapy including conditioning for bone marrow transplant, although experience in critically ill patients is limited. Moreover, several studies have shown that enteral glutamine promotes a down-modulation of the inflammatory cascade resulting in veno-occlusive disease and severe GVHD. Enteral glutamine (30 g/day) has been less studied but one medium sized, randomized trial demonstrated no reduction in mucositis, sepsis, TPN use, time to engraftment, and length of stay. For unclear reasons, glutamine supplementation has been associated with higher mortality rates following autologous bone marrow transplantation, and those receiving methotrexate-GVHD prophylaxis, and may function as a tumor growth factor. At present, in the absence of a contemporaneous large randomized control trial glutamine cannot be recommended for routine use in these settings. Targets of immune-enhancing enteral formulas in the critically ill are presented in Figure 13.3.

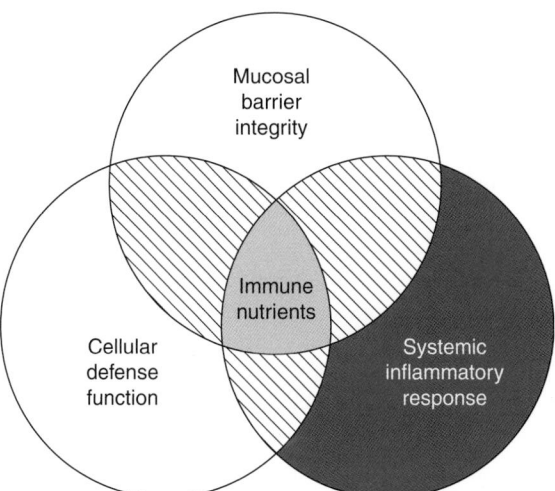

Figure 13.3 Targets of immune-enhancing enteral formulas in the critically ill. (Reproduced from Suchner U, Kuhn KS, Fürst P. The scientific basis of immunonutrition. Proceedings of the Nutrition Society 2000;59(4):553–563, with permission from Cambridge University Press.)

Miscellaneous issues

Probiotics

There is a growing use of probiotics both as preventative and therapeutic adjuncts for infectious diarrhea including *Clostridium difficile* colitis, radiation enteritis, and patients with enteral feeding-associated diarrhea, and to provide intestinal colonization resistance vs hospital acquired, multidrug resistant strains. These preparations usually contain *Lactobacillus*, *Enterococcus*, *Bifidobacterium*, or yeasts such as *Saccharomyces boulardii*. However the safety of probiotic use in immuno-compromised hosts is very questionable as there have been over 80 cases of probiotic-associated infection (usually bloodstream infections) in bone marrow and chemotherapy patients, HIV-1, and organ recipients. Thus probiotic use is not recommended in any category of critically ill immuno-compromised hosts.

Use of enteral tap water for dilution of enteral feeding

Water-borne pathogens are a significant hazard to immuno-compromised hosts. In general it is unnecessary to dilute full strength enteral feedings although it is a common practice to administer "free water" in hypernatremic patients, to flush feeding tubes on a routine basis to prevent clogging, and to administer medications diluted or reconstituted with water. Only purified pyrogen-, preservative-, and microbial-free water (not distilled water) is an acceptable option in critically ill immuno-compromised patients.

Glucose control

Hyperglycemia is very prevalent amongst immuno-compromised critically ill patients resulting in either increased insulin requirements in previously insulin-treated patients or de novo insulin requirements in insulin-naïve patients to maintain tight (80–110 mg/dL) or moderate (110–150 mg/dL) glucose control. The common superimposition of corticosteroid-based immuno-suppression coupled with both critical illness and supplemental continuous nutrition no doubt are all contributory. Parenteral insulin infusions are the gold standard for glucose management. The combined surgical intensive care unit (SICU) and medical intensive care unit (MICU) randomized control data (n = 2748) of conventional versus intensive insulin treatment from Van den Berge et al. showed a mortality benefit in long stay (> 3 days) patients but only included small populations of immuno-compromised patients (hematological and solid organ malignancy, organ transplant) and were not analyzable as a subgroup. Immuno-compromised patients may exhibit a "brittle" pattern of insulin responsiveness due to fluctuations in gastric tolerance, intestinal absorption, corticosteroid dose, and liver function resulting in rapid changes in serum glucose concentration.

Drug–enteral tube interactions

The bioavailability of some medications used in immuno-compromised hosts may be reduced during periods of enteral nutrition. This is less of a problem for drugs (ciclosporin, tacrolimus) which can be monitored by blood levels or for agents with alternative parenteral formulations. Several anti-retroviral drugs (indinavir, ritonavir, atazanavir, daranuvir, zidovudine, didanosine etravine and nevirapine) are rendered unavailable when crushed to administer via enteral feeding tubes. Critically ill HIV patients on previously effective anti-retroviral cocktails need to be switched to alternative agents which remain bio-available during enteral feeding.

Summary points

- Nutritional deficiency states are ubiquitous amongst immuno-compromised patients even prior to medical or surgical conditions which result in critical illness.
- Immuno-compromised patients are a constant concern for clinical care clinicians and the prevention of opportunistic infections has a considered impact on patient's outcomes
- The reduction in infectious complications associated with early initiation of enteral tube feedings versus either no feedings or parenteral nutrition could be an attractive feature in critically ill immuno-compromised hosts.
- Bone marrow recipients represent the greatest challenge in achieving adequate and safe enteral nutrition. In the absence of high level evidence, the decision to use enteral or parenteral or combined support still needs to be individualized on a case-by-case basis.
- Meta-analysis data have shown that enteral formulas supplemented with glutamine, arginine, nucleic acid, omega-3 fatty acids, and antioxidants reduce infectious complications but not overall mortality in a diverse spectrum of critically ill populations.
- Probiotic use is not recommended in any category of critically ill immuno-compromised hosts.

Further reading

Arfons LM, Lazarus HM. Total parenteral nutrition and hematopoietic stem cell transplantation: an expensive placebo? Bone Marrow Transplant 2005;36:281–288.

Heyland DK, Dhaliwal R, Drover JW, et al. Canadian clinical practice guidelines for nutrition support in mechanically ventilated, critically ill adult patients. J Parenter Enter Nutr 2003;27:355–373.

McClave SW, Martindale RG, Vanek VW, et al. Guidelines for the provision and assessment of nutrition support therapy in the adult critically ill patient: Society of Critical Care Medicine (SCCM) and American Society for Parenteral and Enteral Nutrition (A.S.P.E.N.). J Parenteral Enteral Nutr 2009;33:277–316.

Muscaritoli M, Grieco G, Capria S, et al. Nutritional and metabolic support in patients undergoing bone marrow transplantation. Am J Clin Nutr 2002;75:183–190.

Nerad J, Romeyn M, Silverman E, et al. General nutrition management in patients infected with human immunodeficiency virus. Clin Infect Dis 2003;36(Suppl):S52–62.

Nitenberg G, Raynard B. Nutritional support of the cancer patient: issues and dilemmas. Crit Rev Oncol Hematol 2000;34:137–168.

Sanchez AJ, Aranda-Michel J. Nutrition for the liver transplant patient. Liver Transplant 2006;12:1310–1316.

Thompson JL, Duffy J. Nutrition support challenges in hematopoietic stem cell transplant patients. Nutr Clin Pract 2008;5:533–546.

Van den Berghe G, Wilmer A, Milants I, et al. Intensive insulin therapy in mixed medical/surgical intensive care units. Benefit versus harm. Diabetes 2006;55:3151–3159.

Ziegler R. Glutamine supplementation in cancer patients receiving bone marrow transplantation and high dose chemotherapy. J Nutr 2001;131:S2578–S2584.

14

Nutritional support of critically ill cancer patients

Wilson I. Gonsalves and Aminah Jatoi

Introduction

Patients with cancer often appear malnourished: they can present with weight loss, low albumin, a decline in functional status, and a variety of other features consistent with "malnutrition." Importantly, the word "malnutrition" suggests to some that this clinical picture will improve with caloric supplementation. In fact, however, this is often not the case. One of the biggest challenges in cancer care is the realization and acceptance on the part of patients, their families, and even healthcare providers that caloric supplementation, particularly in patients with advanced cancer, can be detrimental and should only be occasionally and judiciously prescribed. The purpose of this chapter is to describe when caloric supplementation appears to be of no value to cancer patients, when it might be of some value, and to provide guidance on how to prescribe it.

Weight loss is a simple, extremely important, and revealing indicator of malnutrition. In a frequently referenced study from the Eastern Cooperative Oncology Group, DeWys and others described outcomes of 3047 cancer patients with weight loss and clearly showed that weight-losing patients were at risk for morbid events that led to a shortened survival. The threshold at which weight loss reached this degree of prognostic significance was > 5%. In other words, regardless of cancer type, tumor burden, and patient performance status, patients who described a weight loss of greater than 5% in the preceding few months lived a shorter life compared to those patients who had reported that they had maintained their weight.

In other settings, many clinicians and researchers have adopted the threshold of 10% to define severe malnutrition in cancer patients. Utilizing this tool to its fullest extent, many clinicians and researchers have come to define a 10% or greater loss of weight as an indicator of severe malnutrition in all patient populations regardless of whether they have cancer or not. The main point here is that weight loss carries a prognostic effect and, under certain

Nutrition in Critical Care, ed. Peter Faber and Mario Siervo. Published by Cambridge University Press. © Cambridge University Press 2014.

circumstances, can trigger some consideration of caloric supplementation to subgroups of cancer patients. Moreover, because cancer therapy is often based on weight, the use of the latter provides a convenient means to assess the nutritional status of a cancer patient in an oncology clinic.

Admittedly, a robust and burgeoning literature describes other methods to assess malnutrition. These other methods include the Patient-Generated Subjective Global Assessment of Nutritional Status as well as a variety of other questionnaires and similar assessment tools. Additionally, body composition assessment methods, such as regional, computerized tomographic scanning of the body (often the L3 lumbar area to capture muscle area), potassium 40 measurement, anthropometry, dual x-ray absorptiometry, and bioelectrical impedance have all been reported as tools for the assessment of malnutrition. Yet others cite the importance of laboratory parameters such as C reactive protein and albumin levels. We believe that all these methods have merit but tend to be of greater value in a clinical trial setting. For purposes of easing patient burden, curtailing time and cost for patients and healthcare providers, and utilizing valuable information that is easily accessible and well-validated, we believe the strongest argument can be made for utilizing weight as an indicator of malnutrition and for making therapeutic decisions based on this parameter.

When and how to intervene

Two interventions are commonly considered in weight-losing, malnourished cancer patients: (1) direct caloric supplementation and (2) nutritional counseling.

Nutritional support

If a cancer patient has lost 10% of his or her weight, should parenteral or enteral supplementation be implemented? The answer to this question is "very likely not." Back in 1989, the American College of Physicians provided a position paper on parenteral nutrition in cancer patients who are receiving chemotherapy. The gist of their statement appears as a direct quote below:

Thus, the routine use of parenteral nutrition for patients undergoing chemotherapy should be strongly discouraged, and, in deciding to use such therapy in individual patients whose malnutrition is judged to be life threatening, physicians should take into account the possible exposure to increased risk.

Now, years later, this statement has not been revised, emphasizing the point that the vast majority of patients, particularly those with advanced cancer, are not candidates for parenteral nutrition or, for that matter, for any effort at aggressive caloric supplementation.

However, under a few circumstances nutritional support might be considered in a cancer setting. First, subgroups of pre-operative cancer patients may derive benefit from it. For example, the Veterans Affairs Cooperative Group study evaluated 395 malnourished cancer patients, 65% of whom had cancer. This thoughtfully conceived clinical trial randomly assigned pre-operative patients to either 7–15 days of total parenteral nutrition with 3 days nutritional support post-operatively versus intravenous therapy without the same caloric value. The bottom line in this trial is that major complications and 90-day mortality were equivalent in the two study arms. However, an *a priori* subgroup analysis revealed that severely malnourished patients (n=24) appeared to have fewer non-infectious complications. A small series of subsequent studies that have looked at pre-operative parenteral nutrition, one in hepatocellular carcinoma patients and one in colorectal/gastric cancer, serve to confirm a potential beneficial role of pre-operative parenteral nutrition in severely malnourished cancer patients. Publication bias that favors reporting only positive studies suggests some caution in drawing firm conclusions, but certainly healthcare providers might consider parenteral nutrition in some groups of malnourished cancer patients who are about to undergo surgery.

Secondly, parenteral nutrition appears to provide benefit to patients at high risk for malnutrition in the setting of high-dose chemotherapy followed by bone marrow transplantation. Justification for this approach comes from Weisdorf and others who randomly assigned 137 such patients to parenteral nutrition versus intravenous fluids. Despite the fact that this study allowed for crossover from the intravenous fluid arm to the parenteral nutrition arm, patients assigned up front to the total parenteral nutrition surprisingly demonstrated an improvement in cancer-free and overall survival rates. Often quoted, this study remains controversial, as results have not been replicated in a study from Charuhas and others. Nonetheless, it appears reasonable that if the mucositis or other chemotherapy-related morbidity is severe to the point that a patient with a potentially curable cancer is unable to eat, resorting to parenteral nutrition during a long period of food deprivation is sensible.

The data that show futility and potential harm associated with feeding most cancer patients are peppered with other studies described above, and, as a result, great confusion seems to abound as to when to provide nutrition support. In our opinion, one must consider the patient's cancer status, the goals of cancer therapy, and the extent or risk of malnutrition in making the decision of whether to provide nutrition support or not. If the likelihood is relatively high that the patient will be cured of his/her cancer or will sustain a long cancer-free period, then it makes sense to provide nutrition support to either treat or stave off malnutrition. If on the other hand, it appears that the patient has widespread, metastatic cancer for which cancer treatment would provide only modest gains, then the benefits of initiating nutritional support appear dubious and should not be prescribed.

Nonetheless, exceptions occur. For example, the Mayo Clinic reviewed its 20-year experience with home parenteral nutrition in incurable cancer patients. This small group of 52 patients comprised 15% of the institution's total number of home parenteral nutrition-treated patients during that given time interval. The median time from starting parenteral nutrition to death was 5 months (range: 1 to 154 months), and 16 patients lived for over a year. The fact that these outliers appear to have done so well underscores again the fact that there are exceptions to every rule. Certainly, it should be emphasized that the patients who did well were in fact the exceptions, as this small group appears to have been cherry-picked based on the clinician's prediction that they likely would live longer than most and hence would benefit from parenteral nutrition. These data are further bolstered by a study from Brard and others which focused on patients with bowel obstructions and again demonstrated the presence of outliers who appeared to benefit from parenteral nutrition. The bottom line is that parenteral nutrition is not for everyone, is not for most cancer patients, but might benefit an extremely small, select group of oncology patients with metastatic cancer.

Although the foregoing applies primarily to total parenteral, the same conclusions pertain to the use of enteral nutrition. The widely taught adage, "If the gut works, use it," might make one wonder if the cautious indications for parenteral nutrition also apply to enteral nutrition. The data to date suggest it does. A recent meta-analysis examined 13 randomized, controlled trials that included 1414 patients; this study looked at the use of enteral nutrition in cancer patients. Importantly, the quality of these studies varied markedly, as manifested by great heterogeneity among trials, thus suggesting that conclusions should be only cautiously put forth. Nonetheless, it appeared that enteral nutrition had some beneficial effect on some aspects of quality of life (emotional functioning, dyspnea, loss of appetite, and global quality of life), but it had no effect on mortality (relative risk = 1.06, 95% CI = 0.92 to 1.22, P = 0.43; I(2) = 0%; P(heterogeneity) = 0.56). Given the highly subjective nature of quality of life assessment, one might conclude that the benefits of enteral nutrition appear nearly as nebulous as those conferred by parenteral nutrition.

If a rational decision is made to prescribe nutrition support, how should it be given? First, it makes sense to utilize the adage referred to earlier, "If the gut works, use it." In effect parenteral nutrition always takes a back seat to enteral nutrition if a patient can tolerate the latter. Second, an estimate of desired caloric content continues to rely on the Harris-Benedict equation that is used in numerous other non-cancer clinical settings to estimate caloric needs. Although this equation has not been specifically validated for cancer patients, it provides good initial estimates of such needs, includes a fudge factor to allow clinical judgment to help with such estimates, and in general gets one started with caloric supplementation with plenty of room to make further adjustments in caloric content over time. Certainly if patients are taking in some of their caloric needs orally or begin to do so, then cutting back on other parenteral feeding is appropriate. Third, the content of parenteral nutrition should include glucose, vitamins and minerals, and fatty acids. A spate of earlier articles raised the question of whether immunonutrition should be prescribed to cancer patients. The latter is defined as the use of specific nutrients, often arginine, glutamine, and omega-3 fatty acids in the nutrition formulation. To date, however, too few high-quality studies have been conducted in cancer patients, a few suggest harm, and in general this approach is expensive. Based on the foregoing, it seems as if immunonutrition should not be part of routine clinical practice among cancer patients.

Nutritional counseling

In the absence of providing enteral or parenteral caloric supplementation to cancer patients, there is another approach that can be used in ill cancer patients: talking with them. Often times, a severe illness that results in an admission to the intensive care unit is a pivotal time in a cancer patient's life, and often times a discussion of end-of-life occurs in that setting. To our knowledge, previous studies have not observed how often the issue of nutrition is a precipitating factor for such discussions, but in our own personal experience, the limitations of providing nutritional support in advanced cancer patients often lead to more extensive end-of-life discussions. These conversations are often difficult, time-consuming, repetitive, but extremely important in terms of helping patients and family members prepare for end-of-life.

Even in advanced cancer patients who are not quite at the very end-of-life but nonetheless struggling to eat, nutritional counseling appears to be a valuable intervention. At least two studies speak to such benefits. Ravasco and others studied 111 colorectal cancer patients before starting radiation. This three-arm study randomized these patients to one of the following arms: (1) dietary counseling on how to help ingest a fairly typical diet versus (2) dietary counseling to help with the intake of protein supplements versus (3) ad libitum intake. Patients who were randomized to either group 1 and 2 described less anorexia, nausea, vomiting, and diarrhea. Importantly, these favorable effects were not short-lived, but in fact sustained as far out as 3 months after radiation.

Secondly, these same investigators found that nutritional counseling helped head and neck cancer patients during radiation. This study included 75 patients who were randomized to one of the following groups: (1) dietary counseling to help ingest regular foods versus (2) dietary counseling in conjunction with nutritional supplements, or (3) ad libitum intake. Important observations include the fact that energy intake was increased with dietary counseling with sustained effects again seen as far out as 3 months after completion of radiation. At 3 months, favorable effects appeared sustained. In general, this group of investigators stands out in favor of dietary counseling among cancer patients, particularly given the positive findings they have generated.

Importantly, in addition to the studies cited above, there have also been negative studies which have shown no detriment but also no benefit from dietary counseling. How might we reconcile the disparate results from these various studies on dietary counseling? In an effort to do so, Halfdanarson and others performed a systematic review and meta-analysis, selecting randomized trials that evaluated dietary counseling in cancer patients and that relied upon a validated quality of life instrument to assess quality of life endpoints. After an exhaustive literature search, these investigators found five such trials that met these investigators' eligibility criteria.

Examined together, the standardized mean difference in quality of life scores among cancer patients who had undergone dietary counseling was 0.56 (95% confidence interval, −0.01–1.14; P = 0.06). These investigators concluded, "Dietary counseling does not appear to improve quality of life significantly in patients with cancer." However, clearly this trend that suggests an improvement in quality of life with dietary counseling suggests that further study of this approach is worthwhile.

In our opinion, it is difficult to dispute the importance of sitting down with a patient and talking with them about their struggles with eating, providing a sympathetic ear, and providing practical advice on how to potentially make things better. Such discussions can often help patients feel less guilty about how they have disappointed family members in not meeting eating goals, and similar guilt among family members who help with food preparation can be lessened in a similar manner. Although the findings from randomized, controlled trials may be generating controversial results, talking with patients and their families about what is bothering them and providing respectful, helpful advice seems nothing short of humane.

Conclusions

Caloric supplementation with enteral or parenteral feeding should be used sparingly in patients with cancer. Although not all studies have been of the highest quality, it appears that cancer patients with severe malnutrition with a great deal of recent weight loss but with some chance of being cured of their cancer or of gaining a highly favorable benefit from cancer therapy, may be candidates for nutritional supplementation. At the same time, for the many cancer patients who have no curative option and who are plagued by weight loss and difficulty eating, dietary counseling may be of some help.

Summary points

- Patients with cancer often appear malnourished.
- Caloric supplementation, particularly in patients with advanced cancer, can be detrimental and should only be occasionally and judiciously prescribed.
- Weight loss is a simple, extremely important, and revealing indicator of malnutrition in cancer patients.
- Enteral and parenteral nutritional support must be individualized and consider the patient's cancer status, the goals of cancer therapy, and the extent or risk of malnutrition in making the decision of whether to provide nutrition support or not.
- Immunonutrition should likely not be part of routine clinical practice among cancer patients.
- Nutritional counseling is an important strategy to improve quality of life in patients not eligible for nutritional supplementation.

Further reading

Baldwin C, Spiro A, Ahern R, Emery PW. Oral nutritional interventions in malnourished patients with cancer: a systematic review and meta-analysis. J Natl Cancer Inst 2012;104:371–385.

Bozzetti F, Gavazzi C, Miceli R, et al. Perioperative total parenteral nutrition in malnourished, gastrointestinal cancer patients: a randomized, clinical trial. J Parenter Enteral Nutr 2000;24:7–14.

Brard L, Weitzen S, Strubel-Lagan SL, et al. The effect of total parenteral nutrition on the survival of terminally ill ovarian cancer patients. Gynecol Oncol 2006;103:176–180.

Charuhas PM, Fosberg KL, Bruemmer B, et al. A double-blind randomized trial comparing outpatient parenteral nutrition with intravenous hydration: effect on resumption of oral intake after marrow transplantation. J Parenter Enteral Nutri 1997;21:157–161.

Dewys WD, Begg C, Lavin PT, et al. Prognostic effect of weight loss prior to chemotherapy in cancer patients. Eastern Cooperative Oncology Group. Am J Med 1980;69:491–497.

Fan ST, Lo CM, Lai EC, et al. Perioperative nutritional support in patients undergoing hepatectomy for hepatocellular carcinoma. N Engl J Med 1994;331:1547–1552.

Halfdanarson TR, Thordardottir E, West CP, Jatoi A. Does dietary counseling improve quality of life in cancer patients? A systematic review and meta-analysis. J Support Oncol 2008;6:234–237.

Hoda D, Jatoi A, Burnes J, et al. Should patients with advanced, incurable cancers ever be sent home with total parenteral nutrition? A single institution's 20-year experience. Cancer 2005;103:863–868.

American College of Physicians. Parenteral nutrition in patients receiving cancer chemotherapy. Ann Intern Med 1989;110:734–736.

The Veterans Affairs Total Parenteral Nutrition Cooperative Study Group. Perioperative total parenteral nutrition in surgical patients. 1991;325:525–532.

Weisdorf SA, Lysne J, Wind D, et al. Positive effect of prophylactic total parenteral nutrition on long-term outcome of bone marrow transplantation. Transplantation 1987;43:833–838.

15

Nutritional support of critically ill patients after gastrointestinal surgery

Shay Nanthakumaran and Jan O. Jansen

Introduction

Critically ill patients who have undergone gastrointestinal surgery have comparable nutritional needs to other critically ill patients. However, there are additional
issues, particularly pertaining to feed delivery, and the presence of malignant
disease, which warrant consideration. The nutritional requirements of patients
who have had gastrointestinal surgery reflect their pre-morbid nutritional state,
chronic health issues, the nature of their underlying gastrointestinal pathology, the
mode of presentation, the type of surgery, and the severity and nature of their
critical illness. This chapter discusses the nutritional management of such patients
in the critical care setting, with particular reference to the type, timing, and route of
nutritional support.

Special considerations in patients undergoing gastrointestinal surgery

Malnutrition is common in hospitalized patients, and especially so in patients
undergoing gastrointestinal surgery. Causes include decreased oral intake,
particularly in the elderly, impaired absorption due to bowel obstruction, previous resections or inflammatory conditions, and the presence of malignant
disease. Nearly half of patients undergoing surgery for gastrointestinal malignancies are malnourished and the proportion is even greater amongst those
with upper gastrointestinal cancers. Malnutrition is associated with impaired
immune function, reduced muscle function, and poor wound healing. This
translates into an increased risk of post-operative complications, length of
hospital stay, and mortality. However, even in the absence of malnutrition,
patients undergoing surgery are exposed to a period of post-operative catabolism and immuno-suppression.

Nutrition in Critical Care, ed. Peter Faber and Mario Siervo. Published by Cambridge University Press. © Cambridge University Press 2014.

Despite obvious conceptual benefits, the provision of nutritional therapy to critically ill surgical patients is poor. Studies have shown that surgical patients are significantly less likely to receive enteral nutrition and more likely to receive parenteral nutrition when compared to medical patients. In addition, surgical patients who receive enteral nutrition start feeding almost a day later than medical patients upon arrival to the critical care unit. Gastrointestinal surgical patients fared even worse than other surgical groups for the above parameters.

Initiation of nutritional therapy after gastrointestinal surgery

Nutritional therapy should be instituted early, and – in the absence of contra-indications – this should take the form of enteral support, even after gastro-intestinal surgery. An obligatory period of starvation was, for many years, an unchallenged part of surgical doctrine, based on the assumption that luminal content may not be tolerated in the presence of an ileus, and that the integrity of anastomoses may be compromised. However, small intestinal motility recovers within hours of surgery, and even in the absence of normal peristalsis a moderate absorptive capacity exists. A recent meta-analysis – although not specifically of studies conducted in the critical care setting – confirmed a significant reduction in infectious complications in patients who were fed within 24 hours of surgery, with no adverse effect on mortality, anastomotic dehiscence, resumption of bowel function, or hospital stay. The evidence is, however, stronger for lower than upper gastrointestinal surgery, although it has been argued that early feeding is probably equally safe and beneficial after hepatic, gastric, and pancreatic resection.

Liver resections do not involve gastrointestinal anastomoses, and post-operative motility problems are rare. Enteral feeding can therefore be commenced immediately. Pancreaticoduodenectomy, in contrast, may be complicated by delayed gastric emptying, and many surgeons therefore delay resumption of oral intake or – in the critical care setting – commencement of enteral nutrition. Experience from higher volume centers, however, suggests that enteral feeding, or oral intake, may be commenced early.

The management of patients undergoing partial or total resection of the stomach has undergone important changes. A recent meta-analysis has shown that there is no need for routine nasogastric or nasojejunal decompression following partial or total gastrectomy. These patients should be allowed to eat, if possible, or fed enterally. Early resumption of oral intake after esophageal resection, however, remains contentious. Gastric conduits, due to their intra-thoracic position and denervation, do not always empty well, resulting in an increased risk of aspiration and subsequent respiratory complications, and nasogastric tube drainage is thus often used to mitigate against these risks. A contrast study is performed 5 days post-operatively, to confirm integrity of the anastomosis and emptying of the gastric tube. If satisfactory, the nasogastric tube can be removed and diet commenced. In order to facilitate calorie delivery during this period, esophagectomy patients should therefore have either an additional nasojejunal feeding tube, or a feeding jejunstomy placed at the time of resection, in which case enteral feeding can be started within hours of surgery. This strategy has been shown to decrease post-operative complications and length of stay, compared with using intravenous fluids alone.

Post-pyloric naso-enteral feed delivery

Even in patients with an anatomically normal upper gastrointestinal tract, intra-gastric feeding, using nasogastric tubes, is associated with complications such as gastroesophageal reflux and aspiration, and delayed gastric emptying, which may result in failure to attain calorific goals. Intuitively, post-pyloric feeding should overcome these issues, but this technique is also associated with problems, in particular the placement and maintenance of nasojejunal tubes.

Meta-analyses comparing gastric and post-pyloric feeding in critically ill patients found no significant difference in the incidence of pneumonia, percentage of calorific goal achieved, mean total energy intake, critical care unit length of stay, aspiration risk or mortality between gastric and post-pyloric feeding groups. The time to start enteral nutrition, however, was significantly longer with post-pyloric feeding. Feeding tube placement difficulties and blockage were significantly less common in the gastric feeding group. It should be noted that the majority of studies in these meta-analyses did not include patients who had undergone major gastrointestinal surgery. These patients are at higher risk of gastroparesis and may be better managed with post-pyloric feeding tubes, perhaps placed intra-operatively although there is inadequate data to confirm this at present.

In summary, although post-pyloric feeding is conceptually attractive, there is no clear evidence that it is advantageous. Although the route chosen is dependent on the clinical setting – such as the presence of an esophagogastric anastomosis – intra-gastric delivery is more physiological and, usually, more convenient than post-pyloric feeding, and thus the preferred route for the initiation of nutritional support.

Surgical access to the gastrointestinal tract

Enteral nutrition in post-operative gastrointestinal surgical patients who are unable to eat, or require supplemental nutrition in addition to their oral intake, can be delivered in a number of ways. These include nasogastric and nasojejunal feeding tubes, as already described, percutaneous gastrostomies and jejunosto-mies, which can be performed with either endoscopic or radiological guidance, and finally surgically placed gastrostomies and jejunostomies.

Nasogastric and nasojejunal feeding tubes are useful in supplementing patients over a short-term period who are unable to physically eat or who require augmen-tation of their oral intake. Unfortunately these tubes are prone to occluding due to their small diameter and are frequently dislodged. Gastrostomies and jejunosto-mies avoid some of these problems.

Feeding jejunostomies are most commonly used following esophagogastric resectional surgery. With an anastomotic leak rate of 10% and a morbidity rate of 40%, even in high volume centers, over 50% of patients developing complications require an alternative to oral feeding beyond 30 days. A recent systematic review combining five randomized controlled and one case-controlled trial evaluating nutritional access routes following esophagectomy concluded that nasojejunal and nasoduodenal tubes were associated with a higher rate of dislodgement and therefore favored the use of feeding jejunostomy. However, feeding jejunostomies are not without complications, with up to a third of patients experiencing complications such as dislodgement or infection. Nevertheless, feeding jejunostomies have become an important adjunct to the post-operative nutritional management of patients with esophageal malignancies.

Patients undergoing lower gastrointestinal surgery rarely require gastrostomy or jejunostomy, as patients are either able and allowed to eat, or can be fed enterally, using a nasogastric or nasojejunal tube, hence avoiding the complications of surgical access. Gastrostomy may, however, have a role in patients who have undergone extensive small bowel resections, where elemental nutrition may need to be considered on a long-term basis.

Post-operative percutaneous gastrostomy placement is sometimes required in patients who have undergone gastrointestinal surgery, and developed complications, either relating to their GI tract, or other systems. Percutaneous placement is associated with a risk of damage to other viscera, and therefore requires a careful assessment of the risks and benefits, and an experienced operator.

In summary, there is little evidence to commend the formation of feeding jejunostomies for short-term nutritional support, as part of the initial surgical management of patients following small bowel and colonic surgery. Nasogastric, or indeed nasojejunal, access is more convenient and probably associated with fewer complications, although there has been no direct comparison. However, routine jejunostomy insertion is recommended in esophagectomy patients to ensure adequate nutrition in patients who develop complications and for those with long-term poor oral intake with associated pre-existing malnutrition.

Enteral nutrition after temporary abdominal closure and continuation of enteral nutrition during scheduled reoperations

Damage control surgery has become an important strategy in the management of patients with abdominal injury and severe physiological derangement. The concept is also increasingly extrapolated to non-trauma emergency gastrointestinal surgery, for example in patients with septic shock due to intra-abdominal sepsis, or those with questionable bowel viability or source control. Damage control surgery usually involves temporary abdominal closure and reoperation, which has brought with it new challenges, including its nutritional management.

Patients who require damage control surgery have accentuated metabolic needs. Classically, however, patients were often not fed enterally until after fascial closure, because exposure of the bowel was thought to result in ileus and intestinal edema, which was felt to be exacerbated by enteral nutrition, thus delaying or preventing fascial closure, or leading to aspiration and pneumonia. The use of parenteral nutrition avoids some of these problems, but may not always be necessary. There is limited evidence, mainly from the trauma setting, that patients with temporary abdominal closures who are managed with early enteral feeding also undergo earlier fascial closure, and have a lower incidence of pneumonia. Unless other contraindications are present, enteral nutrition should therefore be established early in patients with an open abdomen.

The widespread use of damage control surgery has also resulted in a greater number of "relook" or "take-back" operations. If patients are already intubated and ventilated in the critical care unit prior to return to the operating theatre, and there are no plans for extubation immediately after reoperation, the question arises as to whether enteral feeding should be discontinued pre- and intra-operatively. Adherence to standard fasting guidelines intended for elective surgery will result in lengthy interruptions to feeding, and failure to attain nutritional requirements. There is no evidence or guidance to inform a recommendation on this subject. Pre-operative fasting is intended to reduce the risk of aspiration. Unless dislodged during transfer, patients with a cuffed endotracheal tube are arguably not at increased risk of aspiration. It would therefore appear reasonable to continue enteral nutrition.

Immunonutrition

Standard enteral nutrition regimens provide nitrogen and calories. Recently, the concept of providing nutrients which modulate key regulatory pathways has been evaluated, in an attempt to provide immune enhancement, overcome malnutrition- and surgery-related immuno-suppression, and thus prevent complications. To this end, specific amino acids (arginine and glutamine), essential fatty acids (polyunsaturated fatty acids of the n-3 series), and ribonucleic acids in amounts in excess of recommended daily allowances have been used. A number of randomized controlled trials to compare such immunonutrition regimes with standard prescriptions have been performed to determine if immunonutrition has the ability to improve gut function and positively modulate post-operative immuno-suppression and inflammatory response in gastrointestinal surgical patients. These studies have shown a significant enhancement of immune function by increasing lymphocyte and natural killer cell count, polymorphonuclear cell phagocytosis, and immunoglobulin production. In addition, immunonutrition has been shown to improve intestinal microperfusion in gastrointestinal cancer patients.

These in vitro effects have been translated into clinically relevant outcomes, although many of the original studies had conceptual and methodological limitations. Evaluation is complicated by differences in case mix, variations in general feeding strategies (pre-operative, peri-operative, or post-operative), type and dose of immunonutrients, and the use of a variety of outcome measures. An initial meta-analysis included a heterogeneous group of patients ranging from those undergoing major elective gastrointestinal surgery, trauma patients, and other critically ill patients, and showed a reduction in infectious complications and length of hospital stay, but no effect on mortality. The effect was, however, more pronounced in those undergoing major elective gastrointestinal surgery. A more recent meta-analysis focused on this subgroup, and included 2730 patients from 21 original studies. Eleven of these studies comprised only patients undergoing upper gastrointestinal surgery, eight included patients undergoing either upper or lower gastrointestinal surgery, and two included patients undergoing lower gastrointestinal surgery. All except three included patients having cancer surgery. The majority of studies used a combination of arginine, n-3 fatty acids, and RNA as the immunonutrition formula with control groups receiving an isonitrogenous and isocaloric feed. Pre-operative feeding lasted between 5 and 7 days and post-operative feeding started within the first 24 hours and lasted from 3 to 10 days. The prevalence of malnutrition ranged from 8% to 67%. Immunonutrition, whether delivered pre/post- or peri-operatively, significantly reduced post-operative morbidity and length of hospital stay, but again had no effect on mortality. These results suggest that there is a role for immunonutrition in the nutritional management of patients undergoing gastrointestinal surgery, although much work remains to be done.

Summary points

- There is often an unjustified delay in commencing enteral nutrition in surgical patients compared with medical patients.
- After gastrointestinal surgery enteral feeding should be commenced within 24 hours.
- Patients undergoing esophageal resection should have a feeding jejunostomy placed at the time of resection to facilitate early enteral nutrition.
- Patients requiring abdominal reoperations and abdominal closure should be continuously fed to avoid repeated negative energy balance.
- Immunonutrition in gastrointestinal surgery significantly reduces post-operative morbidity and length of hospital stay but not mortality.

Further reading

Bozzetti F, Braga M, Gianotti L, Gavazzi C, Mariani L. Postoperative enteral versus parenteral nutrition in malnourished patients with gastrointestinal cancer: a randomised multicentre trial. Lancet 2001;358:1487–1492.

Cerantola Y, Hubner M, Grass F, Demartines N, Schafer M. Immunonutrition in gastrointestinal surgery. Br J Surg 2011;98:37–48.

Drover JW, Cahill NE, Kutsogiannis J, et al. Nutrition therapy for the critically ill surgical patient: we need to do better! J Parenter Enteral Nutr 2010;34:644–652.

Heyland DK, Dhaliwal R, Drover JW, Gramlich L, Dodek P. Canadian clinical practice guidelines for nutrition support in mechanically ventilated, critically ill adult patients. J Parenter Enteral Nutr 2003;27:355–373.

Ho KM, Dobb GJ, Webb SA. A comparison of early gastric and post-pyloric feeding in critically ill patients: a meta-analysis. Intensive Care Med 2006;32:639–649.

Kreymann KG, Berger MM, Deutz NE, et al. ESPEN Guidelines on Enteral Nutrition: Intensive care. Clin Nutr 2006;25:210–223.

Marik PE, Zaloga GP. Gastric versus post-pyloric feeding: a systematic review. Crit Care 2003;7:R46–51.

Markides GA, Alkhaffaf B, Vickers J. Nutritional access routes following oesophagectomy – a systematic review. Eur J Clin Nutr 2011;65:565–573.

Moore FA, Feliciano DV, Andrassy RJ, et al. Early enteral feeding, compared with parenteral, reduces postoperative septic complications: the results of a meta-analysis. Ann Surg 1992;216:172–183.

Osland E, Yunus RM, Khan S, Memon MA. Early versus traditional postoperative feeding in patients undergoing resectional gastrointestinal surgery: a meta-analysis. J Parenter Enteral Nutr 2011;35:473–487.

Nutritional support of critically ill patients with renal failure

Patricia Wiesen and Jean-Charles Preiser

Introduction

Acute kidney injury (AKI), a common complication occurring during the course of critical illness, is associated with poor patient outcome and increased mortality. Even though the rapid reduction in glomerular filtration rate is the key feature of AKI, metabolic and nutritional consequences are always present. Indeed, both the AKI itself and its treatment by renal replacement therapy (RRT), either continuous or intermittent, alter the metabolism of several macro- and micronutrients. The clinical consequences of the metabolic and nutritional disturbances during RRT are increasingly better understood and differentiated from the AKI-induced alterations.

In order to better understand the nutritional requirements for patients with renal failure this chapter will first examine the metabolic roles of the kidney and the metabolic and nutritional consequences of AKI and RRT.

Metabolic roles of the kidney

The many homeostatic functions of the kidney are summarized in Table 16.1. As a consequence of these numerous functions, the renal metabolic activity is very high: in resting conditions, even though the weight of the kidneys represents only 0.4% of the total body weight, the kidneys account for 10% of whole-body energy expenditure. In case of AKI, the loss of some metabolic functions of the kidney can lead to life-threatening complications (e.g., electrolyte disturbances inducing cardiac arrhythmias) while the loss of other functions only triggers long-term detrimental effects (e.g., lack of erythropoietin synthesis).

Metabolic changes of AKI

Several metabolic alterations observed during AKI can hardly be distinguished from the metabolic changes induced by the critical illness itself, such as an increase

Nutrition in Critical Care, ed. Peter Faber and Mario Siervo. Published by Cambridge University Press. © Cambridge University Press 2014.

Table 16.1 Physiological functions of the kidneys

Plasma concentration by reabsorption and excretion of water
Reabsorption of substances into the blood
Maintenance of salt and ion levels in the blood
Regulation of blood pH by maintenance of the acid–base equilibrium
Excretion of urea and other waste metabolites
Synthesis of erythropoietin
Activation of vitamin D
Gluconeogenesis

in the metabolic rate, stress-related hyperglycemia, increased lipolysis, and protein catabolism. However, the presence of AKI will induce gross or subtle alterations in the metabolism of macro- and micronutrients (vitamins and trace elements) and electrolytes. Importantly, the metabolic changes associated with AKI are proportional to its severity.

Effects of AKI on macronutrients

In terms of energy metabolism, AKI is associated with changes in the pattern of use of energetic substrates. During critical illness, hormonal changes and the inflammatory mediators contribute to an enhanced lipolysis, increased protein turnover and catabolism, insulin resistance, and the preferential use of carbohydrates (over lipids) as energetic substrates. In case of AKI, specific alterations occur:

Carbohydrates

In addition to the typical stress-related hyperglycemia related to insulin resistance and increased endogenous glucose production, the presence of AKI will be associated with a lesser degree of gluconeogenesis (Table 16.1) and with a delayed clearance of glucagon and insulin, thereby leading to high glycemic variability.

Lipids

AKI is associated with increased triglyceride content of the VLDL (very low density lipoprotein) and of the LDL (low density lipoprotein). The total circulating cholesterol, including the HDL-bound fraction, is decreased, as a result of the altered lipolysis.

Furthermore the activity of the peripheral and liver iso-forms of the lipase enzymes are altered during AKI, thereby impairing the lipid clearance by more than 50%. Finally, the mobilization of fat from adipose tissue and the triglyceride clearance are impaired. These factors contribute to the hypertriglyceridemia found during AKI.

Proteins and amino acids

The critical illness-associated intense protein catabolism is typically increased and prolonged in case of AKI. The clearance of most amino acids is increased, up to 1.3–1.8 g/kg/day. Both the insulin resistance and metabolic

Table 16.2 AKI and CRRT influence on micronutrient concentrations

Micronutrients	AKI	CRRT
Trace elements		
Zinc	↘	0 – ↗
Selenium	↘	↘↘
Copper	–	↘↘
Chromium		↘↘
Manganese	↗ (controversial)	↘↘
Iron	↘	↘
Nickel	↘	↗
Vitamins		
Folic acid (B9)	–	↘
Pyridoxal phosphate (B6)	↘	↘
Thiamin (B1)	↘	↘↘
Vitamin C	↘ (controversial)	↘
Vitamin A	↗	–
Vitamin D	↘	–
Vitamin E	↘	↘

Arrows indicate changes in serum concentrations of the trace elements and vitamins.

acidosis typically present during AKI further promote protein catabolism. Amino acid transport across cell membranes is also impaired, inducing an alteration in the physiological handling mechanisms and changes in the compartmentalization of amino acids between cytoplasm and plasma. In case of AKI, the renal steps of synthesis of some amino acids (glutamine, tyrosine, and arginine) are impaired. Therefore, these amino acids become "conditionally" essential in case of AKI.

Effects of AKI on micronutrients

Micronutrients (vitamins and trace elements) play a key role in metabolism, immune function, and antioxidant defense mechanism. Levels of most of these trace elements are usually lower than normal during AKI (due to many coexistent factors in the context of acute phase reaction) leading to variable protein binding, redistribution of elements between plasma and tissues, acute loss of biological fluids, and dilution (edemas). Patients with AKI present an increased oxidative stress, further amplified by the deficiencies in selenium, zinc, and vitamins C and E (Table 16.2).

Acute kidney injury related changes in nutritional status

Nutritional status is an important determinant of outcome. Therefore, the adaptation of nutrition support to the actual patient's status is particularly

Table 16.3 Means for evaluating protein energy wasting and their limitation in the context of AKI

Albumin, pre-albumin, cholesterol	May be lowered by inflammation
Lymphocyte count	Low specificity
Muscle wasting (anthropometry) Body weight	Interference with edema (increasing weight or mask muscle wasting)
Nutritional scoring system (subjective global assessment)	Validated in chronic (not acute) renal failure
Protein catabolic rate	Necessity of dialysate on ultrafiltrate analysis
Energy expenditure (Harris–Benedict/ indirect calorimetry)	Formulas not reliable in critically ill patients Interference with bicarbonate infusion and temperature variation

relevant. The nutritional disorders related to the metabolic response to stress and the magnitude of the waste of lean and fat mass are proportional to the severity of organ dysfunctions, including AKI. In addition, AKI *per se* alters several aspects of the nutritional management. The recognition of AKI-related changes in nutritional status is important to properly manage the nutrition of these patients.

Nutritional assessment

Several indices of nutritional assessment are altered in the presence of AKI, e.g.:
- Fluid overload can increase the weight, and several anthropometrical indices including mid-arm circumference. Likewise, bioimpedance may be unreliable for estimation of body composition.
- Hemodilution can be associated with decreases of the concentrations of several nutritional biomarkers (Table 16.3). The relevance of pre-albumin as a biomarker of the nutritional status is further impaired by the prolongation of its half-life in case of AKI.

Consequences of renal replacement therapy

Metabolic effects of RRT

Several physical and chemical factors are susceptible to influence energy balance during RRT, including the loss of heat, the biocompatibility of membranes, and the buffering agents.

Heat loss

Both continuous renal replacement therapy (CRRT) and intermittent hemodialysis (IHD) induce heat dissipation, thereby decreasing body temperature and basal metabolism. Accordingly, the loss of calories during RRT should be accounted for when estimating the energy balance.

Bio-incompatibility

Used to describe the inflammatory reaction caused by contact between blood and the exogenous material, yielding an increase in energy expenditure. The first generation of cellulose hemofilters was poorly compatible and is no longer used. The biocompatibility of more recent polymers (synthetic membrane such as polysulfone, polyamide, polyacrylonitrile, polymethylmetacrylate) or modified cellulose has been significantly improved.

Buffering agents: citrate, lactate, and acetate

These organic anions are present in the substitution fluids used for CRRT as buffers. Depending on the amount of filtered volume, the body needs to handle defined quantities of bicarbonate, lactate, or citrate. Acetate is no longer used because of its detrimental hemodynamic effects.

Both lactate and citrate can yield energy, as their metabolites can enter the tricarboxylic cycle of Krebs as energetic substrates. The caloric supply by this pathway can be considerable – up to 500 kcal/day with lactate. It is also suggested that substitution fluid containing lactate can increase protein catabolism.

Depending on the composition of the membrane, saturation occurs after 4–8 hours of treatment after which adsorption rapidly decreases.

Nutritional effects of RRT

The loss of electrolytes, amino acids, trace elements, and water-soluble vitamins is significant during RRT (Table 16.2 and Figure 16.1). The magnitude of the loss of nutrients is partially determined by the dose of dialysis (the dose of dialysis is expressed as the kT/V, where k is a constant relying on clearance, T application time, and V total body water). In addition to the dose, anti-coagulation and immobilization can also induce metabolic alterations and the type of RRT will influence the clearance rate of several molecules and nutrients (Figure 16.2). The type of therapy (dialysis or hemofiltration) and duration

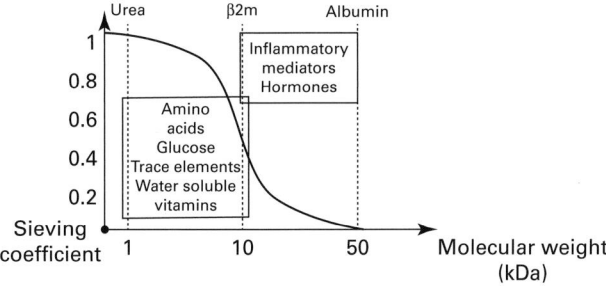

Figure 16.1 **Diagram of the clearance of solutes during RRT. Beta-2m, beta-2-microglobulin.**

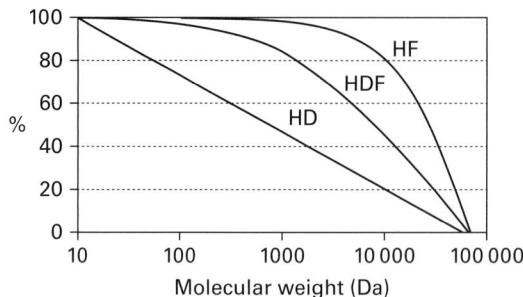

Figure 16.2 **Clearance of solutes during treatment by hemodialysis (HD), HDF (hemodiafiltration) or HF (hemofiltration).**

(continuous or intermittent) further modulates the effects of RRT on the loss of nutrients.

CRRT is commonly preferred over IHD in case of hemodynamic instability, massive fluid overload, and/or cerebral edema. CRRT presents many advantages on intermittent procedures related to the slower fluid shifts and to the more progressive elimination of urea and other small and middle size molecules, including some inflammatory mediators. The methods used for CRRT differ in terms of vascular access, procedure (convection versus diffusion or both), type of membrane, composition, and site of infusion of the substitution fluid. During CVVH (continuous veno-venous hemofiltration), solutes cross the membrane with the solvent by a convective mechanism, following a pressure gradient. The elimination of solutes is proportional to the filtration flow and relies on the membrane permeability. Hence, the CVVH-related physiological and metabolic consequences are dependent on the blood flow, the type of membrane used, the filtration rate, the application time of the treatment, and the anticoagulant used. Every solute with a molecular weight lower than the pore size of the membrane (usually around 20 000 daltons [Da]) will be extracted. Each solute net extraction will depend on its sieving coefficient (Ultrafiltrate/plasmatic concentration) and thus on its clearance (sieving coefficient × ultrafiltration flow). The sieving coefficient of ß2 microglobulin, an intermediate molecular weight (11 000 Da) molecule, is frequently used as a permeability index of a membrane. The physical and chemical properties of the membrane (size of the pores, electrical charge, polymer composition, hydrophilic properties, and thickness) will determine its specific permeability to the different nutrients. The substitution fluid composition resembles the composition of the ultrafiltrate (apart from the buffer and some electrolytes filtered) and the efficacy of the CVVH technique also depends on the site of reinfusion of this substitution fluid (pre- versus post-dilution). Finally, contrasting with intermittent procedures, patients offered CRRT are bedridden – thereby increasing the waste of lean BM.

IHD uses the chemical principle of diffusion (concentration gradient across semi-permeable membrane) where only small molecules can cross the membrane. Hence, the speed of transfer by diffusion will be maximal for small molecules with high plasma concentration. As a result, time of application is lower than with CRRT and losses are limited over time.

Nutritional consequences

The water-soluble substances of low molecular weight weakly bound to proteins will be easily eliminated in proportion to their plasma concentration during convective as well as during diffusive RRT. Any RRT will then induce significant losses of glucose, amino acids, vitamins, and carnitine. Furthermore, RRT exacerbates the protein catabolism and induces the release of oxygen free radicals.

Glucose

Significant gain or loss of glucose can occur, depending on the composition of the substitution fluid or dialysate and on the patient's actual blood glucose concentration. During CVVH, using a substitution fluid without glucose, a glycemia of 100 mg/dL (5.5 mmol/L) with a standard ultrafiltration rate of 2.5 L/hour will result in a daily loss of 60 g of glucose (240 kcal/day) while in the same conditions, a glycemia of 150 mg/dL (8 mmol/L) will be associated with a glucose loss of 90 g/day (360 kcal). In general, glucose-poor substitution fluid solutions are used, resulting in a substantial waste of glucose with a net loss of 40 to 80 g/day according to treatment parameters (filtration flow, pre- versus post-dilution). In these conditions, post-dilution is likely to increase glucose losses as compared with pre-dilution. On the other hand, a net glucose gain is induced by substitution fluid containing 1% glucose or more.

Lipids

Losses due to CRRT are non-significant. There is no need to change the amount or type of lipids of nutrition support.

Peptides and amino acids

All methods of RRT induce activation of protein catabolism through loss of amino acids in the effluent or dialysate and release of cytokines and the consequent inflammatory response. The peptide elimination rate relies on the circulating pool fraction, on turnover, and on the filter sieving coefficient. Protein losses are slightly higher with CRRT techniques based on convection rather than diffusion and can vary from 1.2 to 7.5 g/day. With convective transport, clearance is nearly linear up to the cut off point of the membrane, which corresponds to the pore size (between 20 and 40 kDa). Diffusion also increases protein catabolism and decreases protein synthesis, inducing losses of between 4 and 9 g amino acids and 2 to 3 g of protein.

Because of their small size (mean molecular weight of 145 Da), the sieving coefficient for amino acids is close to one. In case of hemofiltration with post dilution reinfusion of the replacement substitution fluid, the loss of amino acids reaches approximately 0.25 g amino acids per filtered liter (effluent). In consequence, during RRT, relying on the technique and the daily volume used, the amount of amino acids lost is 6 to 15 g/day. Moreover, the rate of elimination of amino acids is also proportional to their plasma concentration (around 10% of the total amount infused is lost). For instance, during CRRT, the clearance of glutamine is higher than the clearance of other amino acids, even if the sieving coefficient is lower than one.

The amount of amino acids to be supplied is around 0.2 g/kg/day to compensate for the losses induced by the treatment. Despite these losses, the serum profile of amino acids does not seem to be modified by CRRT, when low filtration rates are used.

In conclusion, it is proposed to ensure an energetic supply of 25–35 kcal/kg/day with a protein supply of 1.5 to 1.8 g/kg/day.

Electrolytes

Sodium, potassium, calcium, magnesium, and phosphorus are all filtered during RRT. If citrate is used as an anticoagulant in case of CRRT, calcium requirements are higher because calcium is bound to citrate. Recommendations for electrolyte managements for patients with severe AKI on RRT are to adjust intake relying on serum concentration monitoring.

Micronutrients and vitamins

Because trace elements are small molecules, they may be rapidly removed by RRT but on the other hand, dialysate and ultrafiltrate fluid can be "contaminated" with a subsequent supply from the tubing, the membrane, or the substitution fluid. Overall, a significant proportion of the free micronutrients are lost by RRT, resulting in a risk of increased oxidative stress. For instance, selenium losses can vary on a large scale, carrying a risk of clinical deficiency if left untreated. In addition to selenium, other important co-factors of the antioxidant defense mechanisms (manganese, zinc, and vitamin C) are also lost across the CRRT membrane. The type of RRT technique used affects the magnitude of these losses.

Significant waste of water-soluble vitamins is commonly seen during RRT; therefore thiamine, folic acid, and pyridine need to be substituted.

Practical implications for nutrition support

Nutritional recommendations for patients treated by CRRT have been recently updated by a working group of the European Society for Clinical Nutrition and

Metabolism (ESPEN) (available on the website http://www.espen.org/education/espen-guidelines).

In summary, early enteral nutrition (initiated at 24 to 48 hours of admission) with standard formulas rather than those for kidney failure, is recommended in patients with AKI.

CRRT allows unrestricted nutritional support, reaching nutritional targets without the risk of fluid overload and excessive uremia. Nutritional support during CRRT should take into account the extracorporeal losses of nutrients. CRRT using higher effluent rates will accentuate extracorporeal glucose, amino acids, and micronutrient losses. The recommended energy intake is 20–30 kcal/kg/day of non-protein calories (increased in case of burn, trauma, or sepsis but relying on the ideal weight) and should be targeted by indirect calorimetry when available. Calories should be provided as 60–70% carbohydrates and 30–40% lipids.

Protein supply should be 1.5–1.8 g/kg/day during CRRT. A specific glutamine supplementation is recommended since this amino acid becomes conditionally essential and is significantly eliminated by CRRT.

Similarly, the electrolytes that are lacking in the substitution fluid (mostly potassium, phosphorus, magnesium, and sometimes calcium) should be supplemented.

Water-soluble vitamins (vitamins B and C) and the active form of vitamin D should be supplemented to compensate for the losses or the deficient activation while vitamin A supply should be reduced to compensate for the deficient retinol degradation. Nevertheless, recommended vitamin C intake in patients with AKI should be lower than 250 mg/day because of the risk of potentially nephrotoxic secondary oxalosis (Table 16.4).

Finally, the compensation of trace elements lost during CVVH is suggested. The simplest option is to provide a double dose of one of the existing trace element intravenous preparations in case of parenteral nutrition and a single dose when the patients are enterally fed. In all CRRT modalities, selenium and thiamine appear to

Table 16.4 Summary of recommendations (daily doses)

Macronutrients	
Total energy (kcal/kg/day)	25–35
Non-protein energy (kcal/kg/day)	20–30
Proportion of carbohydrates/lipids (%)	60–70/30–40
Protein supply (g/kg/day)	1.5–1.8
Micronutrients	
Vitamin B1 (thiamin) (mg/day)	100 mg
Vitamin C (mg/day)	250 mg
Selenium (µg/day)	100 µg
Folic acid, 1,25 OHvitD	1 mg, 0.25 µg

be the micronutrients at highest risk of depletion. An additional 100 µg (at least 20–60 µg/day) of selenium and 100 mg of thiamine should be intravenously delivered daily while on CRRT.

Conclusion

The frequent use of CRRT has revealed a number of metabolic and nutritional derangements that are not usually associated with either acute kidney injury or with intermittent hemodialysis. In general, standard intake of carbohydrates and and fat, and a slightly increased protein intake are recommended during CRRT, as well as the administration of trace elements and water-soluble vitamins. It should be noted that the type of CRRT procedure, the membrane used, the type of anticoagulation, and the characteristics of the replacement fluid (composition and location of reinfusion) and/or dialysate can all independently influence these recommendations.

Summary points

- Renal failure results in difficult glycemic control, hypertriglyceridemia, and variable impairment of amino acid synthesis.
- Renal replacement therapy can result in large heat loss affecting metabolic rate and energy balance.
- Buffering agents used in renal replacement therapy can add significantly to total daily energy intake and may increase protein catabolism.
- Daily energy intake should be 25 to 35 kcal/day with protein supply of 1.5 to 1.8 g/kg/day.
- Patients with renal failure can experience deficiencies in selenium, zinc, and vitamins C and E, and vitamins and micronutrients should be substituted in patients receiving renal replacement therapy.

Further reading

Berger M, Shenkin A, Revelly JP, et al. Copper, selenium, zinc, and thiamine balances during continuous venovenous hemodiafiltration in critically ill patients. Am J Clin Nutr 2004;80:410–416.

Cano N, Fiaccadori E, Tesinsky P, et al. ESPEN Guidelines on Enteral Nutrition: Adult renal failure. Clin Nutr 2006;25:295–310.

Chioléro R, Berger MM. Nutritional support during renal replacement therapy. Contrib Nephrol 2007;156:267–274.

Druml W. Nutritional management of acute renal failure. J Ren Nutr 2005;15:63–70.

Dungan K, Braithwaite SS, Preiser JC. Stress hyperglycemia. Lancet 2009;373:1798–1807.

Leblanc M, Garred LJ, Cardinal J, et al. Catabolism in critical illness: estimation from urea nitrogen appearance and creatinine production during continuous renal replacement therapy. Am J Kidney Dis 1998;32:444–453.

Leverve XM, Cano NJ. Nutritional management in acute illness and acute kidney insufficiency. Contrib Nephrol 2007;156:112–118.

Schneeweiss B, Graninger W, Stockenhuber F, et al. Energy metabolism in acute and chronic renal failure. Am J Clin Nutr 1990;52:596–601.

Uchino S, Bellomo R, Ronco C. Intermittent versus continuous renal replacement therapy in the ICU: impact on electrolyte and acid-base balance. Intensive Care Med 2001;27:1037–1043.

Wiesen P, Van Overmeire L, Delanaye P, et al. Nutrition disorders during acute renal failure and renal replacement therapy. J Parenter Enteral Nutr 2011;35:217–222.

Nutritional support of critically ill patients with liver and pancreatic failure

Euan Thomson and Alistair Lee

Introduction

Normal liver and pancreatic function is essential to the maintenance of nutritional and metabolic homeostasis. Failure of either organ is associated with high mortality rates, especially in those patients requiring critical care. Good management of these conditions is multi-faceted but, as with all critical illnesses, careful attention to nutritional needs has been demonstrated to improve outcome. The critical care physician needs to be familiar with the nutritional derangements that accompany failure of the liver or pancreas and the specific nutritional interventions that have been demonstrated to improve outcome.

Liver failure

Liver failure is characterized by a loss of normal hepatic function. The condition can be chronic, in which a sustained toxic stimulus leads to progressive hepatocyte damage, inflammation, and ultimately fibrotic change (cirrhosis), or acute, in which an insult causes rapid and widespread hepatocellular death.

Acute liver failure

Acute liver failure is a relatively uncommon condition in which catastrophic hepatocellular damage is associated with marked metabolic upset and multi-organ failure. In the United Kingdom paracetamol intoxication is the leading etiology although in other countries viral hepatitis may be more frequent.

Acute liver failure is categorized by the temporal relationship between onset of jaundice and development of encephalopathy in an individual without pre-existing disease:

Nutrition in Critical Care, ed. Peter Faber and Mario Siervo. Published by Cambridge University Press. © Cambridge University Press 2014.

- Hyper-acute < 7 days
- Acute 8–28 days
- Subacute 4–12 weeks

Hyper-acute liver failure confers a better prognosis than acute or subacute disease. Patients with acute liver failure normally require critical care due to the severity of their primary liver injury.

Pathological consequences of liver failure include cardiovascular collapse, marked coagulopathy, and hepatic encephalopathy; a reversible neuropsychiatric syndrome characterized by progressive obtundation of conscious level.

Chronic liver failure

In the Western World chronic hepatic failure is most commonly due to excessive alcohol consumption. Patients with chronic liver failure often come to the attention of the critical care services when an acute inter-current event, most often systemic or peritoneal infection or gastrointestinal hemorrhage, leads to a rapid deterioration in clinical condition (acute-on-chronic liver failure).

Nutritional assessment in chronic liver failure

Pre-existing malnutrition is almost universal (>90%) in patients with chronic liver disease and cirrhosis admitted to critical care. Malnutrition is multifactorial and is characterized by a decrease in body protein, an increase in total body water, and marked micronutrient and vitamin deficiencies. Malnutrition is associated with an increased incidence of complications and poorer outcomes in both chronic stable disease and acutely deteriorated disease. A variety of tools are available for the assessment of malnutrition but the SGA and anthropometry are commonly used and recommended. Serum albumin should be measured but relatively poorly reflects the severity of protein malnutrition in stable liver disease and even less well so in acute critical illness.

Metabolic consequences of chronic liver failure

Chronic liver failure is a hyper-catabolic, hyper-metabolic state. In those with chronic liver failure resting metabolic rate (RMR) is often 30% greater than in healthy controls. In those with chronic liver failure and associated critical illness energy expenditure may be even higher. Increases in RMR are not universal and ideally indirect calorimetry should be used to accurately quantify energy demands. In the absence of specific measures of RMR guidelines recommend that a calorific supply equal to 1.3 × calculated RMR, based on dry body weight excluding ascitic fluid, can safely be given. The aim should be to provide 25–40 kcal/kg/day for most patients.

Carbohydrate

Hypoglycemia is a common problem in both acute and chronic liver disease and is a result of impaired gluconeogenesis, limited glycogen deposits, and hyper-insulinemia. Hypoglycemia can develop rapidly and even overnight fasting can result in marked hypoglycemia. Intravenous glucose solutions that provide 2–3 g/kg/day of glucose should be used to treat and prevent hypoglycemia. Insulin may be required to prevent hyperglycemia. In total carbohydrate should provide approximately 50–60% of the non-protein calorific requirement of the patient with liver failure.

In patients with chronic liver failure it is essential to ensure adequate replacement of B1 (thiamine) and other B vitamins prior to commencing glucose infusion to prevent the development of Wernicke's encephalopathy.

Protein

The reduced ability of the failing liver to clear metabolites from the portal circulation results in increasing concentrations of toxic nitrogenous compounds entering the systemic circulation. Ammonia is key amongst these and is implicated in the development of encephalopathy. Hyperammonemia is associated with poorer outcome in liver failure. It was previously thought that the omission of protein content from feeding solutions may confer benefit by reducing the plasma concentrations of ammonia and other toxic nitrogenous compounds. Evidence does not, however, support this hypothesis and it is apparent that adequate protein provision can reduce the severity of protein catabolism and improve outcome in liver failure. Current guidelines recommend that 1.2–1.5 g/kg/day of protein or amino acid equivalent be given. Ammonia levels should, however, be measured and feeding regimes adapted to prevent excessive hyperammonemia.

Liver failure is associated with alterations in the plasma protein profile. As liver function declines, aromatic amino acids (AAA) such as tyrosine, phenylalanine, and tryptophan, which are dependent on hepatic metabolism for deamination increase while branched-chain amino acids (BCAA) such as valine, leucine, and isoleucine, which are dependent on muscle metabolism, decline. As BCAA and AAA are dependent on the same transport mechanism to cross the blood–brain barrier an increase in the AAA:BCAA ratio promotes the movement of AAA into the brain. Within the brain AAAs are converted into false neurotransmitters, octopamine, and phenylethanolamine, which contribute to the encephalopathy seen with decompensated and acute liver failure.

Historically, feeds with an increased concentration of branched-chain amino acids have been used in patients with encephalopathy in the hope that they may reduce the severity of the encephalopathy and improve survival. Unfortunately there is limited evidence to support these theories. A previous Cochrane review failed to find any evidence of improvement in outcome using BCAA-enriched feeds although it did find a trend towards improvement in encephalopathy. Current guidelines continue to recommend the use of these feeds but the most recent Cochrane systematic review, which took a more critical look at the methodology of included trials, failed to demonstrate any benefit in patients with hepatic encephalopathy.

Probiotics

In addition to BCAA probiotic feeds have been investigated in patients with liver failure. It was hoped that the use of these feeds would alter the gut flora and reduce the number of intra-luminal ammonia-producing bacteria and subsequently improve encephalopathy. A recent Cochrane systematic review, however, failed to demonstrate any benefit with probiotic use and they are not currently recommended. In the patient with decompensated liver disease and encephalopathy often the most effective intervention is treatment of the precipitating cause.

Lipids

The provision of lipids in both enteral and parenteral nutrition is not contraindicated in liver failure. Lipids should be delivered to provide 40–50% of non-protein calorie supply, approximately 0.8–1.2 g/kg/day. There is some limited evidence that lipid solutions containing increased concentrations of medium-chain triglycerides (n-3) and reduced concentrations of long-chain triglycerides (n-6) may cause less leukocyte suppression and induce less inflammation than standard feeds.

Micronutrients

Deficiencies of micronutrients are common in chronic liver failure. As with all critically ill patients the routine use of supplemental micronutrient preparations is recommended in liver failure. When delivered via the parenteral route care should be taken to avoid excessive supplementation and regular micronutrient screening should be performed.

Route of feeding

No specific advantage to either the enteral or parenteral feeding route has been demonstrated for patients with liver disease although the enteral route is associated with reduced cost and reduced incidence of line-related sepsis when compared to intravenous feeding.

In all patients, attempts should be made to maintain enteral nutrition. In those patients requiring critical care the oral route is frequently unavailable and enteral tube feeding should be commenced. The incidence of gastrointestinal hemorrhage is comparable in both oral and tube-fed patients with esophageal varices. The presence of varices should therefore not be considered a contraindication to nasogastric or nasojejunal tube placement although a fine bore tube should be used to limit esophageal trauma. Percutaneous jejunal feeding tube placement is associated with increased risk in this population due to coagulopathy, portal hypertension, and ascites, and is not recommended.

With no specific contraindications PN should be commenced when either the enteral route in not available, when sufficient calorific content cannot be delivered by the enteral route, or when there is a concern over conscious level and risk of aspiration.

Timing of feeding

Patients with chronic liver disease are frequently malnourished on presentation to the critical care area. In these patients immediate institution of supplemental nutrition is recommended. Attempts should be made to establish enteral nutrition in the first instance and parenteral nutrition instituted if the enteral route is not tolerated. If fasting exceeds 72 hours for any reason then PN should routinely be initiated.

Nutrition in acute liver failure

Acute liver failure (ALF) is a relatively uncommon condition and as such the nutritional aspects of the management of ALF have not been as well studied as chronic liver failure. In a study of 33 European critical care units managing ALF there was a diversity of management strategies. As a rule the nutritional aspects of care will be broadly similar to those with any other critical illness although a number of specific points should be noted:

- All patients with ALF will have a mandatory requirement for intravenous glucose supplementation to prevent hypoglycemia. Infusion rates equivalent to 2–3 g/kg/day will be sufficient to prevent hypoglycemia.
- The majority of patients with acute disease will not have pre-existing dietary deficiencies and therefore the aim of therapy is to maintain nutritional balance in the face of increased metabolic stress. Patients with acute or subacute failure will be at increased risk of protein malnutrition and feeding should commence early. In those with hyper-acute liver failure supplemental nutrition should be commenced if fasting is likely to continue for > 5–7 days.
- As with chronic liver disease the benefit of BCAA-enriched protein supplements is unclear although the majority of critical care units managing patients with ALF continue to use them. Similarly the use of medium-chain triglyceride lipid solutions has some support and may be beneficial.
- Although there is usually no contraindication to enteral nutrition in this patient population the parenteral route is favored by most units due to its reduced aspiration risk in patients with depressed conscious level (Table 17.1).

Pancreatic failure

The pancreas has both endocrine and exocrine functions that are fundamental to normal digestive and metabolic physiology. Endocrine pancreatic functions include the release of insulin, glucagon, and somatostatin and as such it is intimately involved in maintenance of metabolic homeostasis. The exocrine pancreas produces a variety of enzymes including proteases, lipase, and amylase that are secreted into the duodenum to facilitate the digestion of macromolecules into

Table 17.1 Summary of nutritional interventions in liver failure

Route	No specific contraindication to either EN or PN
	Presence of varices is not a contraindication to NG/NJ placement
	Percutaneous feeding tubes not recommended
Timing	High likelihood of pre-existing malnutrition in chronic liver disease – commence feeding early
	In acute hepatic failure commence if fasting > 5–7 days
Calorific requirement	Use indirect calorimetry to measure energy expenditure
	In absence of direct measures assume requirements $1.3 \times REE$ (calculated on euvolemic weight)
	Aim 25–30 kcal/kg/day
Carbohydrate	Carbohydrate should provide 50–60% calorific requirement
	Hypoglycemia common problem
	IV glucose mandatory in acute hepatic failure. Aim 2–3 g/kg/day to prevent & treat hypoglycemia
	Replace thiamine and B vitamins prior to commencing glucose infusion in chronic liver failure
Protein	Protein malnutrition common and associated with poor outcome
	Protein supplementation not associated with worsening of encephalopathy
	Aim to provide 0.8–1.2 g/kg/day
	No evidence that increase in branched-chain amino acid solutions beneficial
Lipid	Lipid supplementation recommended
	Aim to provide 0.8–1.2 g/kg/day
	Medium-chain triglycerides may improve leukocyte function and reduce inflammation
Additional supplements: probiotics, thiamine & B vitamins	No evidence that reduces encephalopathy
	Consider in all patients with chronic liver disease

absorbable entities. Both acute and chronic pancreatic failure has significant nutritional consequences.

Acute pancreatic failure

Incidence and outcome

Acute pancreatitis (AP) is a common condition with an incidence of 0.7 per 1000 population in Western countries and accounts for 11.5 per 1000 hospital admissions. The most frequent etiologies are excess alcohol consumption and biliary cholelithiasis. Although the majority of hospital admissions with acute pancreatitis are mild or moderate in severity, up to 30% of patients with AP will develop severe disease. Severe AP has been estimated to account for 2% of all critical care admissions. Severe AP has an overall mortality of 30% although in those with infected pancreatic necrosis the mortality rate has been reported to be as high as 70%. This contrasts sharply with mild and moderate pancreatitis in which the mortality is less than 1%.

Pathophysiology

Acute pancreatitis is a condition that is characterized by the inappropriate activation of proteolytic enzymes within pancreatic acinar cells leading to autodigestion of cellular components. In mild disease, edema and inflammation are limited to the pancreas itself but in severe disease there is extensive necrosis of the pancreas with spill of proteases into the circulation and activation of multiple inflammatory mediators. The resultant systemic inflammatory response syndrome (SIRS) leads to the development of a multi-organ failure state similar to severe sepsis. Severe pancreatitis can be further complicated by the development of infection of or hemorrhage within the necrotic pancreatic bed. The pathophysiological mechanisms that result in the progression of mild pancreatitis to severe necrotic pancreatitis are not fully understood.

General principles of nutritional management

Patients with mild disease are usually managed in a normal ward setting and will not normally require specific nutritional intervention. The fundamentals of treatment of these patients are adequate analgesia, intravenous fluid hydration, and nil by mouth until pain resolves. Once pain has subsided then oral intake is restarted with a carbohydrate-rich, moderate protein/fat diet progressing to normal diet as tolerated. Patients with moderate disease severity may require enteral nutrition via a nasogastric tube to maintain nutritional status if pain-associated anorexia is prolonged (> 5–7 days).

   Those with severe disease will require critical care admission, aggressive fluid resuscitation and multi-organ support. In these individuals the requirement for specific nutritional support will be almost universal. Good nutritional care is one of the cornerstones of the management of these patients and has been demonstrated to improve outcome.

Parenteral vs enteral feeding

Historically it was thought that continued EN and hence pancreatic exocrine stimulation during AP would perpetuate inflammation and worsen the disease course. Traditional treatment for pancreatitis was therefore to allow for "pancreatic rest" by keeping the patient nil by mouth. Over 30 years ago, however, it was demonstrated that maintaining adequate nutritional input in patients with acute severe pancreatitis conferred a significant survival benefit over no nutritional support and so PN in conjunction with nil by mouth became the treatment of choice. More recent investigation has, however, challenged this treatment paradigm.

The maintenance of a nil by mouth protocol for protracted periods of time in patients with critical illness has been shown to lead to intestinal disuse ischemia and loss of gut mucosa integrity. Loss of normal gut function increases the rate of bacterial translocation and absorption of endotoxins and cytokines from the gut lumen. It is thought that maintaining the enteral route helps to preserve mucosal function and has been shown in animal studies to prevent mucosal bacterial translocation. Additionally EN has been shown, by reducing splanchnic cytokine production, to limit the acute phase response and reduce protein catabolism in acute pancreatitis.

Published data comparing parenteral (PN) with enteral (EN) feeding in acute pancreatitis has recently been subjected to a Cochrane systematic review totalling eight papers including 348 patients. It was demonstrated that, when compared to PN, EN was associated with reduced mortality (relative risk 0.5) and reduced incidence of multi-organ failure (RR 0.55). Benefit of EN over PN was even more marked in those with severe pancreatitis in terms of mortality (RR 0.18) and multi-organ failure (RR 0.46). Across all patients EN was also associated with reduced rates of local and systemic infection, reduced requirement for operative intervention, and shorter length of hospital stay. Additionally enteral nutrition is associated with a lower incidence of hyperglycemia, is cheaper, and reduces the risk of catheter-related blood stream infections when compared to parenteral nutrition.

The benefits of EN over PN are most prominent when EN is commenced early, within 48 hours of hospital admission, and this should be one of the goals of the physician caring for the patient with severe acute pancreatitis (SAP).

Not all patients are tolerant of enteral nutrition. The development of paralytic ileus and/or extrinsic luminal intestinal compression can limit the tolerability of enteral feeding in many patients with severe pancreatitis. If adequate calorific intake cannot be achieved with EN alone then PN should be used to maintain intake. If possible low-dose elemental enteral feeding should be continued in conjunction with parenteral nutrition to maintain intestinal mucosal integrity.

Nasogastric vs nasojejunal route

When compared to gastric feeding, jejunal feeding is associated with reduced pancreatic stimulation and may be better for the patient with acute pancreatitis. Unfortunately nasojejunal tubes are more difficult to place, requiring either endoscopic or radiological guidance and may be impossible to site in patients with intestinal obstruction. Additionally, meta-analyses have not demonstrated a clear benefit of nasojejunal feeding compared with nasogastric delivered nutrition.

Energy expenditure

Severe acute pancreatitis is a multi-system inflammatory condition that is characterized by a hyperdynamic, hyper-metabolic, and hyper-catabolic state. When measured by indirect calorimetry the RMR in patients with this condition is, on average, 1.5 times that estimated by the Harris–Benedict equation. In those with severe acute disease complicated by infected necrosis the RMR may be up to 1.8 times calculated. This is not, however, a universal finding. Only 50% of those with necrotizing pancreatitis have been found to have an elevated RMR, increasing to 80% of those with associated sepsis. It is therefore recommended that all patients with SAP have RMR measured by indirect calorimetry to prevent over- or under-feeding. In the absence of a definitive measure of energy consumption current guidelines suggest 25–35 kcal/kg/day as an appropriate initial target.

Carbohydrate

Alterations in carbohydrate metabolism in pancreatitis are driven by increases in cortisol and catecholamines leading to an increase in gluconeogenesis, increased insulin resistance, and decrease in glucose oxidation. Hyperglycemia, both as a result of these and due to pancreatic islet cell destruction, is common and is a marker of illness severity in those without pre-existing diabetes. Exogenous insulin will be required in up to 80% of patients with severe pancreatitis and should be delivered to maintain normoglycemia.

Despite this, however, adequate provision of carbohydrate is essential in the nutritional management of these patients. Exogenous carbohydrate may reduce gluconeogenesis and therefore limit catabolic protein loss. Carbohydrates, normally delivered as glucose, when delivered by either enteral or intravenous route cause less stimulation of the exocrine pancreas than either lipids or protein. Current recommendations are that 50–70% of daily calorific requirement be provided by carbohydrates.

Protein

Severe acute pancreatitis is associated with a marked catabolic response and significant protein loss. Skeletal muscle catabolism can increase by up to 80% and urinary protein losses of 20–40 g/day are common. Many patients presenting with pancreatitis have pre-existing malnutrition, normally due to chronic alcohol excess. Even in the previously well-nourished patient, however, malnutrition can develop rapidly due to enhanced losses and pain-induced anorexia. Protein energy malnutrition has been associated with up to a 10-fold increase in mortality in acute pancreatitis and therefore one of the primary goals of nutritional therapy in acute pancreatitis is the maintenance of an adequate nitrogen balance. Current guidelines recommend that 1–1.5 g/kg/day of protein be given.

In addition to protein loss SAP is associated with alterations in the plasma amino acid profile, most notably with a reduction in branch-chain and gluconeogenic amino acids (alanine, glutamine, and serine). Although there is evidence to support the use of glutamine supplementation in critically ill patients its use in acute severe pancreatitis specifically has not been well studied. A meta-analysis of the use of PN with glutamine supplementation demonstrated a trend towards improvement in outcome in pancreatitis and the most recent guidelines from the European and American Society of Parenteral and Enteral Nutrition support its use in pancreatitis for patients requiring PN. Daily doses of 0.2–0.4 g/kg L-glutamine are recommended. The use of enteral glutamine supplementation in pancreatitis has not been well studied and is the focus of ongoing research.

Lipids

Abnormalities of lipid profile are both a cause and result of acute pancreatitis. Severe hyperlipidemia is a risk factor for developing acute pancreatitis but acute pancreatitis also results in abnormalities of lipid metabolism. These changes are characterized by increased lipolysis and lipid oxidation and reduced lipid clearance leading to hypertriglyceridemia.

Despite concerns that hyperlipidemia may cause or worsen acute pancreatitis current guidelines support the use of exogenous lipids provided that, ideally, normal triglyceride levels are maintained (< 4 mmol/L) and particularly that hypertriglyceridemia (> 12 mmol/L) is avoided. Triglycerides should be measured regularly and lipid supplementation discontinued if hypertriglyceridemia persists for > 72 hours.

When given parenterally lipids do not cause stimulation of the pancreas and a dose of 0.8–1.5 g/kg/day may be given. If given enterally lipid-containing solutions should ideally be delivered directly into the jejunum via either a nasojejunal tube (NJT) or percutaneous enterojejunal tube (PEJ) as this causes less pancreatic stimulation than nasogastric delivery. When delivered enterally solutions containing medium-chain fatty acids (MCFA) cause less pancreatic stimulation than those containing long-chain fatty acids (LCFA). Ideally solutions with increased MCFA and reduced LCFA should be used although standard feeds can usually be used safely.

Nutritional supplements and micronutrients

A large number of patients with acute pancreatitis will have a history of excessive alcohol intake. They are often deficient in thiamine and B vitamins and consideration should be given to the use of B vitamin and thiamine supplementation in any patient with acute pancreatitis and a history of alcohol excess.

A variety of other agents have been studied as nutritional adjuncts in pancreatitis. Probiotics, which may theoretically help to maintain normal bacterial flora, were associated with an increased mortality in patients with pancreatitis, due in part to an increased incidence of gut ischemia, and are not currently recommended.

As with all critically unwell patients those with severe pancreatitis should be given supplemental daily doses of micronutrients.

Chronic pancreatitis

Chronic pancreatitis is a condition that is managed predominately in the community or ward setting although development of an inter-current illness may result in the admission of the patients to the critical care unit. There are a number of nutritional aspects of this condition that the physician should be aware of.

Chronic pancreatitis is typified by chronic inflammation, fibrosis, and calcification of the pancreas with progressive destruction of pancreatic tissue leading to maldigestion and, when >90% of pancreatic tissue is destroyed, diabetes. Malnutrition in chronic pancreatitis is extremely common either due to the underlying etiology,

Table 17.2 Summary of nutritional interventions in pancreatic failure

Route	Enteral route preferred to parenteral route (reduced incidence of complications)
	Jejunal feeding reduces pancreatic stimulation compared to nasogastric feeding
	Nasogastric feeding is simpler than NJ feeding and may be as effective
	If enteral feeding not tolerated then PN should be commenced in addition to EN
Timing	EN should be commenced within 48 hours of admission
Calorific requirement	Use indirect calorimetry to measure energy expenditure
	Aim 25–30 kcal/kg/day
Carbohydrate	Glucose preferred form of carbohydrate
	May help to reduce protein catabolism
	Avoid hyperglycemia. Exogenous insulin if needed to maintain normoglycemia
	Carbohydrates should provide 50–70% daily calorific requirements
Protein	Sustained nitrogen deficit associated with 10-fold increase in mortality
	Aim to provide 1–1.5 g/kg/day
Lipid	Lipid supplementation recommended
	Aim to provide 0.8–1.2 g/kg/day
	Jejunal or intravenous administration cause least pancreatic stimulation
	Reduced long-chain fatty acid enteral feeding solution may be preferable to normal solutions – less pancreatic stimulation
	Hypertriglyceridemia should be avoided. Monitor triglyceride levels. Aim for triglyceride levels < 4 mmol/L
	Discontinue lipid supplementation if triglyceride levels > 12 mmol/L
Additional supplements: glutamine, probiotics, thiamine & B vitamins	Limited evidence. May be beneficial
	Associated with increased mortality. Not advised
	Consider if history of alcohol excess

approximately 70% of all cases are secondary to excessive alcohol consumption, or develops as a result of the pancreatitis. Up to 50% of patients with chronic pancreatitis have increased REE – even when well. Vitamin and mineral deficiencies are common. In the well patient with chronic pancreatitis the mainstay of treatment is dietary modification and oral pancreatic enzyme supplementation.

In the critically ill patient with chronic pancreatitis consideration should be given to early nutritional support due to the incidence of pre-existing malnutrition. Caution and a high index of suspicion should be employed upon initiation of supplemental nutrition to avoid refeeding syndrome.

Enteral enzyme supplementation should be continued if possible. There is no specific contraindication to NG feeding although this may be precluded by the illness for which they required critical care admission. PN may be required due to illness severity and is not contraindicated. Vitamin, mineral, and enteral pancreatic enzyme supplementation should continue (Table 17.2).

Summary points

- Metabolic rate is increased in patients with chronic liver failure and they should receive 25–40 kcal/kg/day.
- It is essential to ensure adequate replacement of B1 (thiamine) and other B vitamins prior to commencing glucose infusion to prevent the development of Wernicke's encephalopathy.
- Patients should receive intravenous glucose solutions providing 2–3 g/kg/day and in total carbohydrate should provide approximately 50–60% of the non-protein calorific requirement of the patient with liver failure.
- 1.2–1.5 g/kg/day of protein or amino acid equivalent should be given. Feeding regimes may require adaptation to prevent excessive hyperammonemia.
- Enteral feeding regimes are superior in terms of mortality and morbidity compared with parenteral nutrition in patients with pancreatitis.
- Paralytic ileus may require parenteral administration of supplemental nutrition.

Further reading

Al-Omran M, AlBalawi ZH, Tashkandi MF, et al. Enteral versus parenteral nutrition for acute pancreatitis. Cochrane Database Syst Rev 2010;1:CD002837.

Als-Neilsen B, Kortez RL, Gluud LL, et al. Branched-chain amino acids for hepatic encephalopathy. Cochrane Database Syst Rev 2009;2:CD001939.

Córdoba J, López-Hellín J, Planas M, et al. Normal protein diet for episodic hepatic encephalopathy: results of a randomized study. J Hepatol 2004;41:38–43.

Gianotti L, Meier R, Lobo DN, et al. ESPEN Guidelines on parenteral nutrition: pancreas. Clin Nutr 2009;28:428–435.

Mcclave SA, Chang W, Dhaliwal R, et al. Nutrition support in acute pancreatitis: a systematic review of the literature. J Parenter and Enteral Nutr 2006;2:143–156.

McGee RG, Baken A, Wiley K. Probiotics for patients with hepatic encephalopathy. Cochrane Database of Syst Rev 2011;11:CD008716.

Meier R, Ockenga J, Pertkiewicz M, et al. ESPEN Guidelines on enteral nutrition: pancreas. Clin Nutr 2006;25:275–284.

Petrov MS, Correia MITD, Windsor JA. Naso-gastric tube feeding in predicted severe acute pancreatitis. A systematic review of the literature to determine safety and tolerance. J Pancreas 2008;9(4):440–448.

Plauth M, Cabré E, Riggo O, et al. ESPEN Guidelines on enteral nutrition: liver disease. Clin Nutr 2006;25:285–294.

18

Nutritional support and implications for critically ill patients with sepsis

Michael H. Hooper and Paul E. Marik

Introduction

The care of critically ill patients represents a large portion of our healthcare expenditures. In 2005, within the United States, critical care expenses represented 13.4% of all hospital costs and 4% of national healthcare costs. Of all hospital days reported in the United States 15% were days in an intensive care unit. Many critically ill patients have barriers to volitional intake of nutrition, including use of mechanical ventilation, alterations in mental status, and pharyngeal dysmotility. With over 23 million days of critical care annually in the United States, the need for directed administration of nutrition is substantial.

Severe sepsis is a common cause of ICU admission and is often accompanied by respiratory failure, shock, or alterations in mental status. The patients are often not able to eat volitionally, so the need to monitor and directly administer nutrition in these patients is common. In this chapter, we will review the available data on strategies for nutritional support in critically ill patients with a focus and discussion on its application in patients with sepsis.

Sepsis is the result of the systemic inflammatory response to infection. The massive release of pro-inflammatory cytokines leads to widespread inflammation. A variety of mechanistic pathways, including dysregulation of immune function and coagulation, lead to cellular death and end organ damage. In metabolic terms, the acute result of sepsis is a catabolic state and there is significant energy cost to the patient. The treatment of sepsis has traditionally focused on acute, time-sensitive interventions such as administration of antibiotics, addressing the infectious source, hemodynamic monitoring, and resuscitation. Hospitals have dedicated resources towards the institution of system-based reforms to recognize sepsis and deliver acute therapies. Treatments aimed at preventing later complications of critical illness have produced multiple strategies that are applicable to septic patients. Lung protective ventilation, DVT prophylaxis, daily spontaneous breathing trials, interruption of continuous sedation, and early mobilization are

Nutrition in Critical Care, ed. Peter Faber and Mario Siervo. Published by Cambridge University Press. © Cambridge University Press 2014.

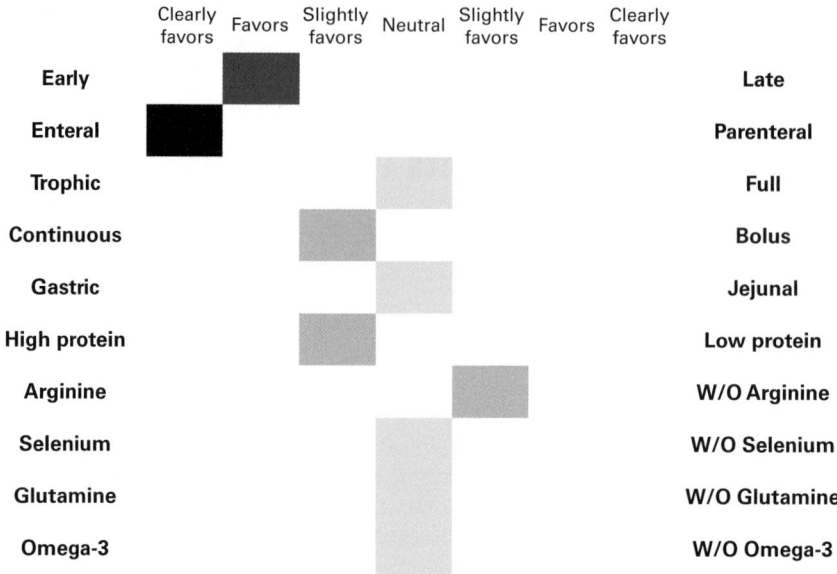

Figure 18.1 Nutritional interventions in sepsis. Certainty of effect on outcomes in non-malnourished patients with sepsis.

examples of strategies which were extensively researched and provided beneficial strategies for supporting critically ill patients. Nutritional support is widely recognized as a necessary part of supportive care in critical illness and research in this field is gradually expanding. As the typical ICU stay of a septic patient is days to weeks, the cumulative energy deficit is extreme and suggests the need for nutritional monitoring and support.

Traditionally, nutritional support has focused on the assumption that striving to meet calculated caloric needs and reach a state of energy equilibrium is paramount. Observation of patients with poor gastrointestinal motility, regurgitation of gastric contents, and aspiration resulted in opinions favoring i.v. administration of nutrition, post-pyloric enteral feeding, meticulous measurement of gastric residuals, and/or various algorithms regarding the rate and timing of enteral feeding administration. Recent data supporting or refuting the many different opinions of practitioners have expanded and significantly changed the evidence-based approach to feeding ICU patients (Figure 18.1).

Which septic patients require nutritional support?

The short answer is that all septic patients who cannot safely maintain volitional oral nutrition require nutritional support. The association between poor nutritional status and poor clinical outcomes has been established in multiple settings and diseases and failure to meet nutritional goals (i.e., underfeeding) is associated with an increased incidence of infection, weakness, duration of mechanical ventilation, and risk of death. These associations alone do not allow the definitive conclusion that nutritional support is beneficial in critically ill patients, but the available evidence suggests that total denial of nutrition for the purposes of a clinical trial would be ethically indefensible. It is accepted practice by multiple professional societies that nutritional support should be provided to the critically ill.

What is the ideal route for delivery of nutritional support?

Enteral vs parenteral

When tolerated, the use of enteral nutrition as the primary source of nutritional support is widely accepted among healthcare professionals. This is reflected in guidelines from the American Society of Parenteral and Enteral Nutrition (ASPEN), the European Society of Parenteral and Enteral Nutrition (ESPEN), and the Canadian Critical Care Practice Guidelines (CCCPG). Controversy emerges when patients have a relative contraindication to enteral nutrition or when patients are unable to "tolerate" enteral nutrition. Specifically, controversy exists in three areas:

- What constitutes a contraindication to enteral nutrition?
- When should parenteral nutrition be started if enteral nutrition cannot be given?
- When should parenteral nutrition be used to supplement "inadequate" enteral nutrition?

Perceived contraindications to enteral nutrition are numerous and deserve discussion. Few anecdotal contraindications are evidence-based. The most common reasons for withholding enteral feeding are either concern of aspiration risk or convenience during complicated patient care. While the goal of preventing aspiration is laudable, the evidence suggests that unnecessarily withholding enteral feeds leads to underfeeding, which may lead to significant complications and morbidity. Temporary disruption of feeding for diagnostic testing, procedures, and other aspects of ICU care may be unavoidable, but every institution should revamp protocols and education to minimize these disruptions.

Of particular concern to many physicians is enterally feeding patients with hemodynamic instability or shock who may have increased gastric reflux or decreased bowel mobility. An increased risk of aspiration pneumonia is perceived to exist in patients with shock. Reports of ischemic bowel in hemodynamically compromised patients receiving enteral nutrition through jejunostomy tubes have also been published in the surgical critical care literature. These concerns have led some physicians to declare shock as a relative contraindication to enteral nutrition. The ASPEN guidelines from 2009 include a general recommendation to withhold enteral nutrition in the setting of "hemodynamic compromise" until the patient is fully resuscitated and/or stable. Notably, this recommendation is "Grade E" and based on expert opinion. Review of the literature does not support the conjecture that enteral feedings in patients with vasopressor dependent shock results in individual adverse events or generally worse outcomes. Multiple published clinical trials evaluating early enteral nutrition in critically ill patients have included patients with septic shock. Bowel ischemia or infarctions are not reported in these clinical trials.

A paucity of data limits our ability to definitively state what conditions are contraindications to enteral nutrition. Complete bowel obstruction and short-bowel syndrome are accepted contraindications. Many other common reasons for avoiding enteral nutrition, such as high residuals, history of aspiration, respiratory distress, hemodynamic instability, or upcoming procedures are either unsupported by literature or only transient reasons to withhold nutrition. Our opinion is that enteral nutrition is very rarely contraindicated in septic patients. Low volume feeds should generally be attempted. If concerns of tolerance develop, enteral feeds may be stopped, but the patient should be continually rechallenged rather than abandoning attempts at enteral nutrition. Withholding of enteral feeds for routine intensive care or procedures should be minimized.

The guidelines of the ESPEN recommend initiation of parenteral nutrition within 48 hours after ICU admission if enteral feeds are inadequate. The American (ASPEN) and Canadian (CCCPG) guidelines recommend early enteral nutrition but suggest that parenteral nutrition may be delayed for 7 days in patients who are not malnourished at baseline. A recent multi-center, randomized, controlled trial compared the strategies of "early" parenteral nutrition vs "late" parenteral nutrition to provide supplemental nutrition to patients failing to meet enteral nutrition targets. The data from this trial showed superiority of the "late" parenteral nutrition group with earlier ICU and hospital discharge, less infections, and less complications during their hospitalization. This trial did not include a group of patients without any parenteral nutrition, so does not allow a comparison to enteral nutrition alone. However, the data do support delay in the initiation of parenteral nutrition in critically ill patients.

Gastric vs jejunal

Jejunal feeding has been compared with gastric feeding in multiple randomized trials not specific to sepsis. These trials did not show clear superiority of one method or the other in terms of volume of feeds administered during the trials. Three studies showed a decreased rate of pneumonia with jejunal feeding, but without other outcome improvements. Mortality and hospital length are similar among patients receiving gastric or jejunal delivery of enteral nutrition. Two separate meta-analyses (2003 and 2006) have shown no benefit to jejunal feedings.

The current evidence does not support a general recommendation for jejunal feeding, but if jejunal feeding can be *easily* delivered then it is reasonable to consider in patients at high risk for aspiration or those with GI intolerance. Risky interventions or procedures should not routinely be performed to ensure jejunal feeding.

When should nutritional support be initiated?

Multiple randomized studies suggest that early introduction of enteral nutrition is beneficial in terms of infectious complications. In a meta-analysis pooling RCTs in several specific populations (surgery, trauma, head injury, burns, general medical), early enteral nutrition was correlated with less infectious complications and decreased length of stay. A recently published systematic review of the literature found one trial in which early enteral nutrition led to improved survival, while 15 trials led to decreased length of stay. A single study on early administration (day 1) of full enteral nutrition versus later administration of full enteral nutrition (day 5) showed an increased rate of infectious complications and longer lengths of stay in the group with early initiation. This single outlying study may be the result of significant underfeeding as the daily caloric intake in the late feeding group was roughly 100 kcal/day with only 5 g of daily protein. The early feeding group received an average of ~500 kcal/day which is roughly equivalent to "trophic" feeding in more recent trials. The current position of multiple professional societies is that early initiation of feeding in critically ill patients is necessary and appropriate in most critically ill patients. The initial volume, caloric goals, and content of initial feeding are further discussed below.

How frequently should nutritional support be administered?

Administration of enteral feeding is performed either by intermittent bolus feeds or by slow continuous administration. Intermittent bolus feeding is generally not recommended for post-pyloric or small bowel feeding, but may be considered in gastric feeding. Little data is available comparing the two methods in critical illness or sepsis. Five randomized studies exist in the literature and did not report a difference in mortality, but fewer interruptions and greater volume of feeding is reported with continuous infusions. Continuous feeding is also preferred in nurse polling due to improved workflow.

Data specific to sepsis are not available, but extrapolating from the critical care literature, continuous feeding appears advantageous while the patient remains in a critical care environment. The lack of significant outcome data should give clinicians confidence that continuous feeds may be interrupted or switched to intermittent boluses in certain circumstances. Continuous feeding regimens should not interfere with early mobilization, spontaneous awakening trials, spontaneous breathing trials, or necessary procedures or interventions.

What is the ideal caloric intake and what proportion should be carbohydrates, fat, and protein?

The ideal caloric intake for a septic patient is not known. Observational data have suggested that drastic underfeeding or overfeeding may negatively impact patient outcomes. An interaction with severity of illness seems to exist, which complicates the task of forming guidelines for caloric intake.

Randomized controlled data from the EDEN trial have provided some high-quality data on which to base decision-making for enteral nutrition in the early phase of critical illness. Eighty percent of the population in EDEN was considered septic, so the data provide specific guidance in caring for the septic patient. In the EDEN trial, essentially equivalent patient outcomes were observed when comparing a "full" feeding group (25–30 kcal/kg/day) with a "trophic" feeding group (10–20 kcal/hour) during the initial 6 days of critical care for ARDS. The EDEN protocol resulted in caloric intake of ~ 1300 kcal/day in the "full" feeding group and ~ 400 kcal/day in the "trophic" feeding group. Both groups received "full" feeding after the initial 6 days and all patients were fed the majority of their calories continuously. The equivalent results in the EDEN trial do not inform clinicians exactly how to proceed with the nutritional support of every patient, but does suggest that a wide range of caloric intake in the early phase of sepsis is acceptable for guidelines and protocols. Patients with severe malnutrition, severe neuromuscular disease, and/or refractory shock were among the patients excluded from enrollment. The EDEN trial may not be applicable to these subsets of septic patients. Given the lack of difference in outcomes, patients with significant nutritional deficits may deserve an earlier transition to "full" calorie feeds that approximate their caloric expenditures. In patients with GI intolerance or severe hemodynamic instability, "trophic" calorie feeds may be the most appropriate method for early feeding. Nutritional requirements in the late/recovery phase of critical illness tend to be less controversial, with most experts agreeing that administering caloric intake in an effort to match energy requirements is an acceptable goal. Target values of caloric goals are ~ 25–30 kcal/kg/day. Figure 18.2 shows acceptable caloric goals in typical septic patients.

The formulation of feeding in terms of proteins, carbohydrates, and fat has relevance in terms of outcomes in sepsis. Concerns of differences in absorption, CO_2 production, immune function, and muscular reconstitution have led to various opinions and investigations comparing different formulations of enteral and parenteral nutrition.

Protein catabolism has been observed in septic patients and neuromuscular weakness is a significant morbidity for survivors of sepsis. Neuromuscular weakness during critical illness is substantial and predictive of mortality. Prolonged neuromuscular dysfunction and weakness has significant consequences for rehabilitation and needs at discharge. Observational data have demonstrated improved nitrogen balance and minimization of protein loss in patients who receive aggressive protein supplementation. Observational data also show that adequate delivery of

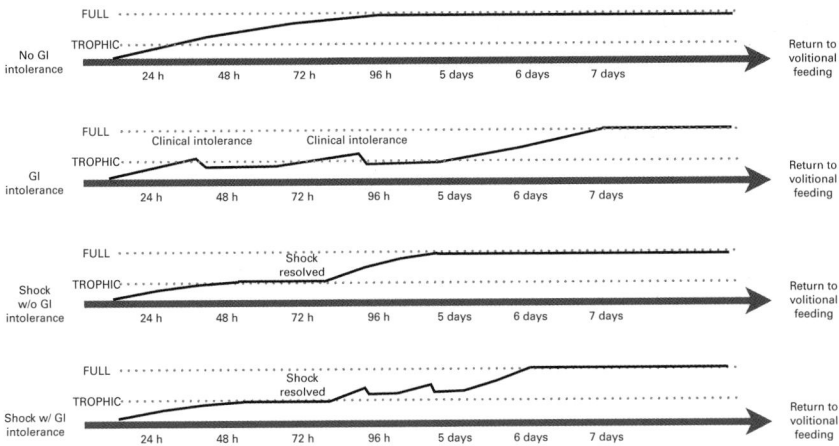

Figure 18.2 Acceptable caloric goals in septic patients, for patients with/without shock or GI intolerance.

protein in nutritional support is associated with improved survival in critically ill patients. Large randomized, controlled trials are lacking. Without RCTs demonstrating improved outcomes, the recommendation for aggressive protein supplementation (approximately 1.2–1.5 g/kg) is based on observational studies and expert opinion. Protein loss is still experienced at that level of supplementation, but evidence does not exist showing larger amounts of protein administration leads to less protein loss or better outcomes. Extrapolation of this recommendation to septic patients seems appropriate given the significant protein loss and weakness experienced in septic patients.

Data on the proper amounts of carbohydrate and fat administration are scarce. As previously mentioned, overfeeding is associated with worse outcomes and should be avoided, regardless of the proportion of calories derived from carbohydrates or fats. Hyperlipidemia, fatty liver, cholestasis, steatohepatitis, and poor immune function are reported as complications of lipid emulsions in parenteral nutrition. A study in trauma patients found worse outcomes with lipid emulsions in TPN versus TPN without lipid emulsions. Another small study in the general hospital population showed no difference between hypocaloric, lipid-free TPN vs eucaloric TPN with lipids. Similar concerns regarding lipids are not reported with enteral nutrition. The shift towards lipid metabolism in the setting of acute illness suggests that calories from fat are important when administering nutritional support, but due to the potential complications of i.v. administration, it is likely that the ideal proportions of carbohydrates and fats for enteral delivery of nutrition are different from those in parenteral delivery of nutrition. There is not widespread agreement on the ideal proportion of carbohydrates and lipids that should be incorporated into parenteral or enteral nutritional support. An individualized approach to each patient is prudent.

Are there other supplements or components that should be included?

In patients with overwhelming infection (i.e., sepsis), the question arises of whether or not nutritional supplements may potentiate or modulate immune function and influence outcomes. Multiple clinical investigations have sought to partially answer this question by assessing the effect of various supplements thought promising based on basic science data or theory. In general, the trials of immune-modulating nutritional supplements have been done in heterogeneous populations, with varying formulations, and have produced mixed results. Numerous nutrients have been proposed and tested, but we will review data on only the most widely available or researched dietary supplements in sepsis.

Arginine

The interaction of arginine with key pathophysiological mechanisms in sepsis as well as its role in establishing a positive nitrogen balance suggests this amino acid could be a potential beneficial additive to nutritional therapy in septic patients, whether in the early or late phases of illness. Arginine is consumed in a normal diet, but is largely endogenously produced via the citrulline intestinal–renal axis. Plasma levels of arginine are noted to be decreased in sepsis due to both increased plasma clearance of arginine and deficiencies in *de novo* production. Lower plasma levels of arginine predict worse outcomes. Arginine is the substrate for nitric oxide (NO) production by NO synthase and is thought to play a key role in systemic and local vascular dilatation and flow in sepsis. The complex pathophysiology of sepsis makes it difficult to state that NO production is either good or bad in sepsis as it may be detrimental when administered systemically, but beneficial if active in specific vascular beds. An attempt to use i.v. administration of an arginine analog in patients with sepsis perhaps demonstrated this complexity as shock reversal was expedited, but mortality was increased. Nutritional investigations were also attempted with supplementation of enteral feeds. Unfortunately, the available trials have been inconsistent in terms of the formulation of the feedings or other supplements included. A meta-analysis by Heyland failed to show a significant effect of arginine in sepsis. Multiple professional societies have cautioned against the use of arginine in patients with severe sepsis. We agree that the current body of data does not support arginine supplementation in sepsis; however, more rigorous investigations with adequate controls could produce different results, particularly in the late (anabolic) phases of sepsis when muscle regeneration and nitrogen balance are increasingly important and systemic vasodilatation has resolved.

Glutamine

In the absence of critical illness, glutamine is an abundant amino acid with large amounts of muscular stores. Depletion of glutamine during critical illness was first reported by Vinnars et al. nearly 40 years ago and subsequently confirmed in multiple separate observations. Observational data have demonstrated that lower glutamine levels are associated with increased mortality in critically ill patients. Determining whether or not glutamine depletion is a marker of severe illness or a cause of poor outcome has been the goal of numerous investigations.

Proposed mechanisms by which glutamine deficiency may lead to worse outcomes in sepsis are varied. Detrimental variation in immune function is commonly hypothesized and supported by multiple observations. Proper functioning of macrophages, lymphocytes, and neutrophils requires glutamine and low levels of glutamine are associated with lymphocyte dysfunction. Increased susceptibility to oxidative stress has also been proposed. Glutathione is an important endogenous scavenger of reactive oxygen species, and glutamine is an important substrate for glutathione. Glutamine depletion is associated with glutathione depletion, thus accumulating oxidative stress in muscle or other tissues depleted of glutathione may contribute to many complications of critical illness. Loss of integrity of gut mucosa is yet another mechanism by which glutamine deficiency may affect critically ill patients and predispose patients to bacterial translocation and recurrent sepsis.

Multiple controlled studies of glutamine have been attempted in critically ill populations. A 2002 meta-analysis suggested an overall benefit to glutamine administration, but the results have been mixed based on the route of glutamine delivery or the studied population. Enterally delivered glutamine in burn and trauma populations has resulted in less infectious complications and has resulted in decreased mortality in a single unpublished trial of burn patients. Results of enterally delivered glutamine in general ICU populations have been less promising with no consistent improvement in patient outcomes by enteral delivery. Parenteral delivery of glutamine has yielded mixed results with some trials demonstrating benefit but two larger, more recent trials that failed to show a significant benefit. Harm from glutamine administration has not been demonstrated. We do not recommend its use in general ICU patients or septic patients, but do not find evidence that its use would be harmful. In burn and trauma populations or in patients receiving parenteral nutrition, supplementation with glutamine should be considered.

Selenium

Data from human studies show significant changes in both humoral and cell-mediated immunity with chronic supplementation with selenium. Protection against hepatitis B infection with selenium supplementation supports this observation. Selenium deficiency has been associated with increased virulence of Coxsackie virus and increased mortality in HIV infection. However, one large (150 patient) randomized, controlled study of selenium in patients with sepsis failed to show any effect on inflammatory markers, mortality, or other outcomes. Another large (502 patient) trial in a general population of critically ill patients also failed to show any improvement in patient outcomes. Selenium does appear to produce measurable effects on humoral and cell-mediated immunity, but the clinical impact of this is unclear. The current data on selenium supplementation in patients with sepsis suggest that it is ineffective and should not be widely used.

Omega-3 fatty acids, GLA, and antioxidants

The inflammatory properties of eicosanoids liberated during the systemic inflammation of sepsis are determined by their membrane phospholipid composition. Omega-3 (n-3) fatty acids favor production of trienoic prostaglandins and series 5 leukotrienes that have significant anti-inflammatory properties. In studies of patients with acute lung injury, levels of n-3 fatty acids are as low as 6% of normal. One omega-6 fatty acid, gamma-linolenic acid (GLA), has also shown promise as potentiating an anti-inflammatory pathway with data suggesting a reduction in pro-inflammatory, arachidonic acid-derived eicosanoids. Three randomized controlled trials in patients with acute lung injury showed that administration of an enteral formula enriched in n-3 fatty acids, GLA, and antioxidants improved respiratory physiology compared to an enteral formula without these supplements. Decreased time or need for mechanical ventilation was seen in all three of these studies with decreased ICU and LOS (length of hospital stay) reported in two studies. A 1000-patient study was planned by the NHLBI ARDS Clinical Trials Network, called the OMEGA trial. This study was planned as a 2×2 factorial design with the EDEN trial which compared "trophic" and "full" feeding strategies in patients with ARDS. In the OMEGA protocol, either 240 mL of n-3, GLA, antioxidant-enriched nutrients or 240 mL of an isocaloric control were given twice daily as an enteral bolus. Patients were randomized to "trophic" or "full" feedings for the EDEN protocol and calories obtained via the OMEGA protocol were subtracted from daily feeding goals in the EDEN trial. This was continued for 21 days or until cessation of mechanical ventilation. After 272 enrolled patients, the OMEGA trial was stopped by *a priori* stopping rules for futility. Patients in the n-3 enriched group had significantly fewer ventilator-free days (primary outcome) and a trend toward increased 60-day mortality (26.6% vs 16.3%, P=0.54).

   The results of the OMEGA trial are contradictory to the previously referenced randomized controlled trials and contradictory to a wealth of basic science literature that predicts a beneficial, anti-inflammatory effect from an n-3, GLA, antioxidant feeding regimen. Criticisms of the OMEGA trial focus on the low protein administered as well as the potential for interaction of effects in the 2×2 factorial design. Patients randomized to both "trophic" and n-3 enriched arms received a very small amount of protein in the initial week of critical illness. All patients in the n-3 enriched arm received less protein than controls. N-3 fatty acid-enriched formulas have previously been recommended by multiple professional societies for patients with sepsis or ARDS. The results of the OMEGA trial will likely alter those recommendations and result in considerable variations in practice among clinicians. The current state of the literature does not support a firm recommendation to continue n-3 fatty acid supplementation for patients with sepsis.

Conclusions

Recent high-quality clinical trials have allowed for more specific recommendations on how to provide nutritional support to patients presenting with sepsis. Enteral feeding is the preferred route and ideally is the only route utilized for nutritional support unless patients have very significant GI tract abnormalities. The use of parenteral nutrition should be reserved for patients who have not tolerated enteral feeding for extended periods of time. During the first week of sepsis, use of "trickle" or "trophic" low calorie feeding is likely equivalent (in terms of outcomes) to more aggressive feeding aimed at matching the patient's caloric expenditures. Caloric goals in the first week of sepsis should be higher for malnourished patients. In most patients, jejunal feeding does not offer any significant advantage to gastric feeding and should not be prescribed routinely. Continuous administration of enteral feeding is likely preferable to intermittent bolus feeding, but may be tailored to individual patient needs.

The ideal proportion of protein:carbohydrate:fat is unclear, but observational data and expert opinion support early and continued goals of 1.2–1.5 g/kg/day of protein supplementation. The data on effects from additional supplements aimed at immune modulation are mixed. Arginine and selenium are likely not beneficial and should not be routinely supplemented in septic patients. Glutamine is likely beneficial in patients receiving TPN and trauma and burn populations. Enteral supplementation with glutamine in septic patients is not generally recommended. Randomized, controlled trials examining the effects of n-3 fatty acids in critically ill patients have produced contradictory results. Differences in methodologies may explain why results have not been consistent.

Summary points

- The patients are often not able to eat volitionally and the cumulative energy deficit is extreme which suggest the need for nutritional monitoring and support.
- Enteral nutrition is very rarely contraindicated in septic patients. Low volume feeds should generally be attempted. Withholding of enteral feeds for routine intensive care or procedures should be minimized.
- It is reasonable to consider jejunal feeding in patients at high risk for aspiration or those with GI intolerance.
- Continuous feeding appears advantageous while the patient remains in a critical care environment.
- The ideal caloric intake for a septic patient is not known. Observational data have suggested that drastic underfeeding or overfeeding may negatively impact patient outcomes.
- Protein catabolism has been observed in septic patients and neuromuscular weakness is a significant morbidity for survivors of sepsis.

- Overfeeding is associated with worse outcomes and should be avoided, regardless of the proportion of calories derived from carbohydrates or fats. There is not widespread agreement on the ideal proportion of carbohydrates and lipids that should be incorporated into parenteral or enteral nutritional support.
- The current body of data does not support n-3 fatty acid, arginine, glutamine, and selenium supplementation in sepsis.

Further reading

Casaer MP, Mesotten D, Hermans G, et al. Early versus late parenteral nutrition in critically ill adults. New Engl J Med 2011;365(6):506–517.

Davis JS, Anstey NM. Is plasma arginine concentration decreased in patients with sepsis? A systematic review and meta-analysis*. Crit Care Med 2011;39(2):380–385.

Freund H, Atamian S, Holroyde J, Fischer JE. Plasma amino acids as predictors of the severity and outcome of sepsis. Ann Surg 1979;190(5):571–576.

Gianotti L, Alexander JW, Gennari R, Pyles T, Babcock GF. Oral glutamine decreases bacterial translocation and improves survival in experimental gut-origin sepsis. J Parenter Enteral Nutr 1995;19(1):69–74.

Heyland DK, Novak F, Drover JW, et al. Should immunonutrition become routine in critically ill patients? A systematic review of the evidence. JAMA 2001;286(8):944–953.

Ho KM, Dobb GJ, Webb SAR. A comparison of early gastric and post-pyloric feeding in critically ill patients: a meta-analysis. Intensive Care Med 2006;32(5):639–649.

Kao CC, Bandi V, Guntupalli KK, et al. Arginine, citrulline and nitric oxide metabolism in sepsis. Clin Sci 2009;117(1):23–30.

Kreymann KG, Berger MM, Deutz NEP, et al. ESPEN Guidelines on Enteral Nutrition: Intensive care. Clin Nutr 2006;25(2):210–223.

Long CL, Schiller WR, Blakemore WS, et al. Muscle protein catabolism in the septic patient as measured by 3-methylhistidine excretion. Am J Clin Nutr 1977;30(8):1349–1352.

Marik PE, Zaloga GP. Early enteral nutrition in acutely ill patients: a systematic review. Crit Care Med 2001;29(12):2264–2270.

McClave SA, Martindale RG, Vanek VW, et al. Guidelines for the Provision and Assessment of Nutrition Support Therapy in the Adult Critically Ill Patient: Society of Critical Care Medicine (SCCM) and American Society for Parenteral and Enteral Nutrition (A.S.P.E.N.). J Parenter Enteral Nutr 2009;33(3):277–316.

Novak F, Heyland DK, Avenell A, Drover JW, Su X. Glutamine supplementation in serious illness: a systematic review of the evidence. Crit Care Med 2002;30(9):2022–2029.

Pontes-Arruda A, Martins LF, de Lima SM, et al. Enteral nutrition with eicosapentaenoic acid, γ-linolenic acid and antioxidants in the early treatment of sepsis: results from a multicenter, prospective, randomized, double-blinded, controlled study: the INTERSEPT study. Crit Care 2011;15(3):R144.

Shaw JH, Wildbore M, Wolfe RR. Whole body protein kinetics in severely septic patients. The response to glucose infusion and total parenteral nutrition. Ann Surg 1987;205 (3):288–294.

Singer P, Berger MM, Van den Berghe G, et al. ESPEN Guidelines on Parenteral Nutrition: Intensive care. Clin Nutr 2009;28(4):387–400.

Villet S, Chiolero RL, Bollmann MD, et al. Negative impact of hypocaloric feeding and energy balance on clinical outcome in ICU patients. Clin Nutr 2005;24(4):502–509.

19

Nutrition in cardiac intensive care

Peter McCanny, Danny Collins, and Andrew A. Klein

Introduction

Cardiac intensive care most frequently cares for patients following cardiac surgery. Tight glycemic control and nutritional support are fundamental aspects of the care of such patients, and together they form a type of metabolic support, just as important as all the other complex and technological organ support modalities that may be required.

Nutritional screening and assessment

Nutritional screening and assessment are part of the nutritional support process, with screening required to determine if the patient is malnourished or at risk of malnutrition. A basic form of screening should be carried out in all patients admitted for cardiac surgery, and more detailed assessment reserved for those identified to be at greatest risk of malnourishment. This may apply especially to elderly patients, patients with chronic heart failure or 'cardiac cachexia', especially when they present for more advanced support, such as mechanical circulatory device implantation or transplantation. Two nutritional screening instruments commonly applied to hospitalized adult patients are the Nutritional Risk Screening (NRS-2002), endorsed by the ESPEN, and the Malnutrition Universal Screening Tool (MUST), developed by the British Association for Parenteral and Enteral Nutrition (BAPEN).

A comprehensive nutritional assessment in critically ill adult patients involves a detailed assessment requiring time and expertise by a trained professional in nutritional assessment and should be done within 24 hours of intensive care admission. A nutritionally focused physical exam is an excellent tool to help evaluate nutritional status.

It is composed of a number of components.

1. Measurement of nutrient balance; factors that may lead to malnutrition and nutritional prognosis of patient:

Nutrition in Critical Care, ed. Peter Faber and Mario Siervo. Published by Cambridge University Press. © Cambridge University Press 2014.

- A review of past medical and surgical history and current illness
- Overall organ function or failures
- Catabolic stress (fever, sepsis, infections, procedures)
- Medications which may decrease nutrient absorption (phenytoin, oral iron), increase nutrient excretion (diuretics), or cause glucose intolerance (corticosteroids)
- Hemodynamic status and inotropic requirements
- Blood electrolytes, biochemical profiles for organ function indices
- Blood triglycerides
- Blood concentration of vitamins/minerals if indicated

2. Measurement of body composition:
   - Obtain body weight history
   - Calculate current body weight; calculate body weight loss/gain from usual body weight over the last few months
   - Calculate current body weight as % of ideal body weight (IBW)
     % of IBW=weight/IBW × 100
     80% to 90%=mild malnutrition
     70% to 79%=moderate malnutrition
     < 70%=severe malnutrition

Serial measurements should be taken to record any change. Factors indicative of malnutrition include involuntary weight loss or gain of $\geq 10\%$ of usual body weight within 6 months or $\geq 5\%$ of usual body weight in 1 month:

- Determine BMI. In adults a BMI of less than 15 kg/m^2 is associated with a significant increase in morbidity
- Evidence of micronutrient deficiencies
- Wound healing
- Fluid balance
- Evaluation of anthropometric data

3. Evaluation of gastrointestinal function:
   - Tolerance of enteral nutrition; presence of ileus, large gastric aspirates
   - Short-bowel syndrome (< 200 cm functional small bowel)
   - Vomiting (> 5 days)
   - Diarrhea (> 500 mL/24 hours × 2 days)
   - Recent abdominal surgery

4. Estimate protein, calorie and micronutrient requirements.

5. Choose route (enteral/parenteral or mixture) for nutrient delivery. The enteral route is always the preferred route if feasible. Parenteral nutrition should be used when the gastrointestinal tract is not functional or cannot be accessed and in patients who cannot be adequately nourished by EN.

Relevance of BMI in cardiothoracic intensive care

Body mass index (either too low or high) has a significant effect on survival in the lung (single or double lung) and cardiac transplant population.

The recent International Society for Heart and Lung Transplantation listing criteria for heart transplantation state that a BMI < 30 kg/m^2 or percent ideal body weight < 140% should be achieved, before listing for cardiac transplantation. An analysis of 19 593 orthotopic heart transplant recipients over a 10-year period identified underweight (BMI < 18.5 kg/m^2) or obesity (BMI > 35 kg/m^2) as having significantly higher morbidity and mortality than other groups.

One retrospective study of 11 411 lung transplant patients showed that the BMI of recipients had a significant effect on first year survival. Mortality was higher in underweight (BMI < 18.5 kg/m^2), overweight (BMI 25–29.9 kg/m^2), and obese (BMI > 30 kg/m^2) lung transplant patients than normal weight controls. Other nutritional risk factors for increased ICU mortality in lung transplant recipients are BMI below the 25th percentile and low pre-transplant pre-albumin levels; there have been no observed differences in relation to serum albumin levels and mortality. In the cystic fibrosis population, nutritional status may be optimized by percutaneous gastrotomy placement while on the pre-transplant waiting list.

Although extremes of BMI are associated with decreased survival after cardiac and lung transplantation, higher BMI does not seem to adversely affect outcome survival after left ventricular assist device implantation (LVAD). This is important because LVADs are used as destination therapy for advanced heart failure patients who are not candidates for transplantation.

Nutritional support in critically ill cardiac patients

The main purpose of nutritional support in cardiac intensive care is to minimize negative energy and protein balance. Negative energy balance has been shown to correlate with an increasing number of complications. The total daily energy requirement of critically ill patients rarely exceeds 35 kcal/kg ideal body weight and the main requirements and distribution on macronutrients do not differ from other critically ill patients.

Carbohydrates

Carbohydrates should provide 50–60% of total calories during nutritional support. In enteral feeding, a variety of carbohydrates such as polysaccharides, oligosaccharides, sucrose, and dextrose can be used. In parenteral nutrition, glucose is the only carbohydrate in common use.

The recommended minimal and maximal doses of glucose are 2 g/kg/day and 6 g/kg/day respectively.

Lipids

Lipids should cover 20–40% of total calories. Corn and soybean oils are commonly used lipid sources for enteral polymeric formulas. For parenteral nutrition, in the

United States only soybean oil-based emulsions are available. In European countries, fish oil, mixtures of olive and soybean oils, medium-chain triglyceride-soybean oil mixtures, and combinations of these oils are approved for use in parenteral nutrition. The recommended minimal and maximal doses of lipid emulsion are 0.5 g/kg/day and 1.5 g/kg/day respectively.

Protein

Protein provides 15–25% of total energy in enteral polymeric formulas. The proteins may be in their original natural forms (milk, egg protein) or as protein isolates separated from original foods. In PN, an amino acid solution is administered which provides all nine essential amino acids and eight non-essential amino acids. The recommended daily dose of protein is 1.2 to 1.5 g/kg/day.

Vitamins

Vitamins are essential micronutrients in both health and disease. Critical illness can affect vitamin metabolism in a number of ways:

- Increased production of reactive oxygen species in illness will lead to increased utilization of antioxidant vitamins such as vitamins C and E.
- The hyper-metabolic rate associated with critical illness leads to an increased requirement, especially of water-soluble vitamins which function as co-factors in metabolic pathways.
- There is altered distribution of vitamins in the body with levels falling due to a fall in carrier proteins. There may also be increased loss of water-soluble vitamins during dialysis.

Trace elements

Both PN and EN nutrition should provide adequate amounts of zinc, copper, selenium, iron, molybdenum, chromium, cobalt, iodide, manganese, fluoride, and vitamin B12. Assessment of trace status during critical illness is difficult as plasma concentrations are a poor reflection of tissue status.

Fluid and electrolyte requirements

Requirements will be influenced by the underlying condition of the patient. Fluid requirements can be calculated roughly as 30–35 mL/kg/24 hours plus 500 mL/24 hours per degree of pyrexia. Electrolyte requirements need to be balanced against excess losses (e.g., attributable to fistulas or diarrhea) or underlying medical conditions such as cardiac or renal impairment. A summary of electrolyte requirements is presented in Table 19.1.

Table 19.1 Summary of adult requirements for electrolytes

Electrolyte	Enteral nutrition	Parenteral nutrition
Sodium	60–100 mmol/day or 1 mmol/kg	80–100 mmol/day
Potassium	50–100 mmol/day or 1 mmol/kg	60–150 mmol/day
Calcium	20 mmol/day or 0.2 mmol/kg	2.5–5 mmol/day
Magnesium	10–18 mmol/day or 0.2 mmol/kg	8–12 mmol/day
Phosphate	20–40 mmol/day or 0.3 mmol/kg	15–30 mmol/day

Nutritional support in mechanically ventilated, critically ill adult patients

Cardiothoracic surgery or illness initiates a catabolic response which can be modified by treating or moderating its underlying cause, but the catabolic response cannot be reversed by nutritional support. Nutritional support can compensate for the negative energy and protein balance and minimize or reduce tissue loss, until the convalescence phase begins. Negative energy balance has been shown to correlate with an increasing number of complications, but not mortality.

The best available evidence to date does not support the practice of permissive underfeeding and current models suggest that providing more than two-thirds of prescribed calories (ideally > 85%) is associated with reduced mortality. Critically ill patients receive, on average, only 40% to 50% of their prescribed nutritional requirements.

Current American, European, and Canadian guidelines are intended for surgical and medical critically ill patients who are expected to require an ICU stay of > 2 days. Therefore they are applicable for those cardiothoracic intensive care patients who have a complicated post-operative course requiring an extended intensive care stay.

Enteral nutrition

First establish if there is no contraindication to enteral nutrition. Contraindications are:
- Intestinal obstruction or ileus.
- Intractable vomiting/diarrhea refractory to medical management.
- Severe short-bowel syndrome (less than 200 cm small bowel remaining).
- Distal high-output (> 500 cc) fistulas (too distal to bypass with feeding tube, e.g., colovaginal fistula).
- Severe GI bleed.
- Severe GI malabsorption (graft-versus-host disease/radiation enteritis/chemo-therapeutic mucositis/severe IBD).

- Inability to gain access to GI tract.
- Severe shock.
- Intestinal ischemia.
- Severe intra-abdominal sepsis.
- Abdominal compartment syndrome.

If there are no contraindications to EN then:

1. EN is the preferred route for feeding over PN for patients requiring nutritional support therapy.
2. Early EN (within 24–48 hours following admission to ICU) is recommended in critically ill patients.
3. The feed rate should be advanced towards the target rate over the next 48–72 hours, using a feeding protocol that incorporates pro-kinetics at initiation and a higher threshold of gastric residual volumes (250 mL) and the early use of post-pyloric feeding tubes.
4. In critically ill patients with feed intolerance, a recommendation is made for the use of metoclopramide as a pro-motility agent. The recommendation does not extend to erythromycin due to associated safety concerns.
5. Small bowel feeds should be considered in critically ill patients who repeatedly demonstrate high gastric residual volumes and are not tolerating adequate amounts of EN delivered into the stomach.
6. There is insufficient data to support the use of enteral glutamine in enterally fed critically ill patients (with the exception of burn and trauma patients).
7. Critically ill patients receiving enteral nutrition should have the head of the bed elevated to 45 degrees.

In clinical practice, most critically ill patients are given 22–25 kcal/kg/day to avoid the metabolic complications of overfeeding.

Effects of enteral feeding on mechanically ventilated patients on inotropic support

Being mechanically ventilated and on inotropes is not a contraindication to enteral feeding. In 2010, a large multi-center retrospective study looked at non-surgical, mechanically ventilated, inotropic-dependent patients, and classified them as to whether they were fed within the first 48 hours (early group) or after 48 hours (late group). After propensity score matching, the early group had a lower ICU (22.5% vs 28.3%; P=0.03) and hospital mortality (34% vs 44%; P < 0.001) compared to the late group. A subgroup analysis demonstrated that the beneficial effect was more evident in the sickest patients, such as those on multiple vasopressors compared to those only on one vasopressor, and in those patients without early improvement, that is, patients who required vasopressors for more than 2 days, with a significant survival advantage (odds ratio 0.36). Early enteral feeding on an intention to treat analysis was associated with a 30% to 35% decreased risk of death with no evidence of harm.

However, being on vasopressors is a risk factor for GI intolerance, so a prudent approach is advocated:

- Prioritize resuscitation.
- Start "trickle" feeds: 10–20 mL/hour within the first 24–48 hours after ICU admission.
- Maintain this rate for 24 hours with appropriate frequent assessments.
- Monitor the patient for intolerance (abdominal distension, rising lactate, large gastric residual volumes).
- If the patient is tolerating that rate and clinical condition is improving, start progressively increasing the feeding rate to target rate.

Vigilance is warranted in the post-operative cardiothoracic surgical population where there is an incidence of mesenteric ischemia of 0.1%–0.5%. Risk factors include prolonged cardiopulmonary bypass, use of an intra-aortic balloon pump, advanced age, and emergency surgery. The diagnosis is difficult to make and a high index of suspicion is indicated in a scenario of stalled or deteriorating post-operative clinical course and persistent intolerance to enteral feed (exhibited by large gastric aspirates), particularly combined with abdominal distension.

Parenteral (total or supplemental) nutrition

1. All patients not expected to be on normal nutrition within 3 days should receive PN within 24 to 48 hours if EN is contraindicated or if they cannot tolerate EN (2009 European Guidelines).
2. The American and Canadian guidelines recommend that PN should not be started in critically ill patients until all strategies to maximize EN delivery have been attempted, and that PN should be delayed in the post-operative period for 5–7 days.
3. In instances where PN is prescribed to critically ill patients, parenteral supplementation with glutamine is strongly recommended.
4. All patients receiving less than their targeted enteral feeding after 2 days should be considered for supplementary PN (2009 European Guidelines); overfeeding should be avoided.
5. In patients receiving PN, repeat periodic attempts should be made to initiate EN. As tolerance of EN improves, the amount of calories supplied by PN should be reduced proportionately. PN should not be terminated until $\geq 60\%$ of target energy requirements are being delivered by the enteral route.
6. Carbohydrate should be administered at a minimal rate of 2 g/kg/day.
7. Intravenous lipid should be administered as an emulsion at a rate of 0.7 g/kg to 1.5 g/kg over 12–24 hours.
8. In PN, a balanced amino acid solution should be infused at 1.3–1.5 g/kg/ideal body weight; it should be comprised of 0.2–0.4 g/kg/day of L-glutamine accompanied by an adequate energy supply.

As parenterally fed patients must metabolize or excrete all infused nutrients, the composition of nutritional formulas should be adapted to nutritional requirements, metabolic capacity, metabolic disturbances, and co-existing deficiencies or overdosing.

There is no reliable method for measuring a patient's precise requirements and metabolic capability, in order to avoid potentially severe metabolic disturbances and refeeding syndrome. It is better to initiate parenteral energy intake at an amount lower than estimated and to increase the nutritional regime slowly depending on the patient's metabolic response. The provision of one-third to one-half of nutritional requirements should suffice initially and be increased to target gradually over a few days, depending on the patient's metabolic response.

Timing of supplemental parenteral nutrition in the critically ill: early versus late debate

Timing of supplemental parenteral nutrition in the ICU is an area of ongoing controversy. The American guidelines advocate continued underfeeding with EN solely for up to 7–10 days prior to the addition of supplemental PN, in contrast to the early addition of PN (within 24–48 hours) in the European guidelines. Advocates for early supplemental PN refer to data that shows that a cumulative energy deficit is associated with adverse outcomes in critically ill patients, with a cumulative energy balance of –10 000 kcal associated with increased mortality and morbidity. Opponents of early supplemental PN refer to the literature demonstrating increased adverse events in patients who receive PN at any point during their ICU admission. The EpaNIC study (Early versus Late Parenteral Nutrition in Critically Ill Adults) was an unblinded, multi-center trial that was an attempt to compare the effects of early initiation of PN versus late PN. The primary outcome measured was ICU length of stay, which was a day shorter in the late PN group (3 vs 4 days). Infections developed in 22.8% of patients in the late PN group, compared with 26.2% in the early PN group (P=0.008). Mortality rates were similar in both groups, both during their ICU stay and at 90 days. This study, however, involved the administration of a large glucose load parenterally (1200 kcal as a 20% glucose solution), which would not be considered standard ICU practice today.

The EpaNIC study consisted of 90% surgical patients, predominantly cardiac, 59% admitted electively for a relatively short period of time. The majority of patients were not malnourished, as evidenced by a BMI between 20 and 30 in 75% of the study patients, raising the issue as to whether they needed supplemental PN at all, especially in the early group. Further studies are ongoing to clarify the issue of early versus late PN in high-risk patients.

Blood glucose control

Hyperglycemia is common in critically ill patients in cardiac intensive care, with approximately 90% of patients developing blood glucose concentrations > 6.1 mmol/L. Hyperglycemia is independently associated with increased mortality. The first randomized controlled trial to compare intensive insulin therapy (IIT) with conventional insulin therapy was a landmark trial published in 2001, conducted by Van Den Berghe et al. in Leuven, Belgium. They studied surgical (mainly cardiac) patients, and reported a 34% reduction in in-hospital mortality. A follow-up study on medical ICU patients published in 2006 failed to show a reduction in mortality with IIT.

Three subsequent multi-center, randomized, controlled trials examining the effect of IIT in critically ill patients have failed to replicate the findings of the 2001 Leuven trial. The 2009 Normo-glycemia in Intensive Care Evaluation-Survival Using Glucose Algorithm Regulation (NICE-SUGAR) showed increased mortality with this approach. Similarly, the 2008 Efficacy of Volume Substitution and Insulin Therapy in Severe Sepsis (VISEP) and the 2009 Glucocontrol trials failed to demonstrate any benefit of IIT over conventional insulin therapy.

The current evidence does not support the widespread adoption of intensive glucose control in critically ill cardiac patients; however glucose control should not be ignored, due to its effect on mortality. The optimal blood glucose concentration for cardiac patients remains unclear. Current recommendations are:

- Blood glucose concentrations should be monitored closely in all critically ill patients.
- Insulin treatment should be commenced when glucose concentrations exceed 10 mmol/L.
- The target blood glucose concentration should generally be between 8 and 10 mmol/L.

Refeeding syndrome

This is a potentially lethal complication of refeeding (EN or PN) in patients who are malnourished from whatever cause. It is caused by too rapid refeeding with carbohydrates leading to electrolyte and pathophysiological disturbances of a potentially life-threatening nature.

Its principal manifestations are:

- Hypokalemia due to rapid cellular uptake of potassium as glucose and amino acids are taken for the synthesis of glycogen and amino acids.
- Hypophosphatemia due to increased phosphorylation of glucose and synthesis of adenosine triphosphate.
- Hypomagnesemia due to increased cellular uptake.
- Rapid depletion of thiamine, leading to Wernicke's encephalopathy and/or cardiomyopathy and also lactic acidosis.
- Salt and water retention leading to heart failure, which may be exacerbated by concomitant thiamine deficiency.

It is best prevented by identifying at risk patients. Restoring circulatory volume and increasing calorie intake slowly over a period of 1–10 days are required in such patients, particularly when malnourishment has been severe and prolonged. The aim is to start at a low level of calorie provision (e.g., 10 kcal/kg/day measured body mass; not IBW). Fluids may need to be restricted to achieve an even balance, and sodium should be restricted to < 1 mmol/kg/day. Electrolytes and vitamins (200% recommended daily intake, thiamine 200–300 mg i.v.) should be replaced before starting feeding, and should be measured 4–6 hourly during the initial stages of feeding. Typical daily electrolyte requirements are:

- Potassium 1–2.2 mmol/kg/day.
- Magnesium 0.3–0.4 mmol/kg/day.
- Phosphate 0.5–0.8 mmol/kg/day.

Conclusion

Further studies are required to allow us to optimize nutritional and intensive metabolic support in cardiothoracic critical care. We need to know more about glycemic control, including individual variability, diurnal variation, and the effects of operative control on the critical care course. It is possible that new technology, especially catheter systems and closed-loop feedback, will allow fine-tuned, individually tailored control in the future, and thus improve outcomes further.

Summary points

- Under- and overweight heart transplant recipients have increased mortality.
- Enteral glutamine supplementation does not improve outcomes in critically ill cardiac patients.
- To assess feeding tolerance enteral nutrition should be increased slowly in ventilated patients on inotropic support.
- When enteral feeding is not tolerated it remains unclear if parenteral nutrition should be started late (5–7 days) or early (1–2 days) after ICU admission.

Further reading

Allen JG, Arnaoutakis GJ, Weiss ES, et al. The impact of recipient body mass index on survival after lung transplantation. J Heart Lung Transplant 2010;29:1026–1033.

Casaer MP, Mesotten D, Hermans GW, et al. Early versus late parenteral nutrition in critically ill adults. N Engl J Med 2011;365:506–517.

Heyland DK, Cahill N, Day AG. Optimal amount of calories for critically ill patients: depends on how you slice the cake! Crit Care Med 2011;39:2619–2626.

Khalid I, Doshi P, DiGiovine B. Early enteral nutrition and outcomes of critically ill patients treated with vasopressors and mechanical ventilation. Am J Crit Care 2010;19:261–268.

Kondrup J, Rasmussen H, Hamberg O, Stanga Z. Nutritional risk screening: a new method based on analysis of controlled clinical trials. Clin Nutr 2002;22:321–336.

Martindale RG, McClave SA, Vanek VW, et al. Guidelines for the provision and assessment of nutrition support therapy in the adult critically ill patient: Society of Critical Care Medicine and American Society for Parenteral and Enteral Nutrition: Executive Summary. Crit Care Med 2009;37:1757–1761.

Moritoki EGI, Finfer S, Bellomo R. Glycemic control in the ICU. Chest 2011;140: 212–220.

Russo MJ, Hong KN, Davies RR, et al. The effect of body mass index on survival following heart transplantation: do outcomes support consensus guidelines? Ann Surg 2010;251:144–152.

Singer P, Berger M, Van den Berghe G, et al. ESPEN Guidelines on Parenteral Nutrition: Intensive Care. Clin Nutr 2009;28:387–400.

Singer P, Anbar R, Cohen J, et al. The tight calorie control study (TICACOS): a prospective, randomized, controlled pilot study of nutritional support in critically ill patients. Int Care Med 2011;37:601–609.

Villet S, Chiolero RL, Bollman MD et al. Negative impact of hypocaloric feeding and energy balance on clinical outcome in ICU patients. Clin Nutr 2005;24:502–509.

20

Nutritional support of critically ill patients with respiratory disorders

Krista L. Turner

Introduction

As one of the defining parameters of critical illness, pulmonary failure demands that the practitioner carefully design a nutrition program to improve care and avoid complications. Administration of macronutrients and micronutrients can affect pulmonary function in several ways: via muscle function, CO_2 elaboration, and immune modulation via inflammatory factors. Fluid balance, electrolyte homeostasis, and acid–base balance also influence pulmonary function and should be considered in the nutrition plan. Pulmonary-specific formulas and immunonutrition should be tailored to each patient based on co-morbid conditions and level of evidence for their use.

Respiratory disorders in critical care

Respiratory disorders that require critical care management consist primarily of acute respiratory insufficiency and chronic ventilator dependence. The acuity and severity of disease can originate from a variety of causes. Neurological injury, alteration in mental status, or airway obstruction often require endotracheal intubation for airway protection. Cases of acute respiratory insufficiency may arise secondarily from heart failure, pulmonary embolism, pulmonary hypertension, or other problems related to pulmonary vasculature. Acute exacerbations of chronic pulmonary diseases may also require short-term stay in an ICU setting. An appropriately designed nutrition strategy should focus on safely feeding the ventilated patient based on the instigating cause of pulmonary failure.

Acute lung injury/acute respiratory distress syndrome

One particular subset of pulmonary disease has recently become the focus of specialized nutrition support. Acute lung injury or acute respiratory distress

Nutrition in Critical Care, ed. Peter Faber and Mario Siervo. Published by Cambridge University Press. © Cambridge University Press 2014.

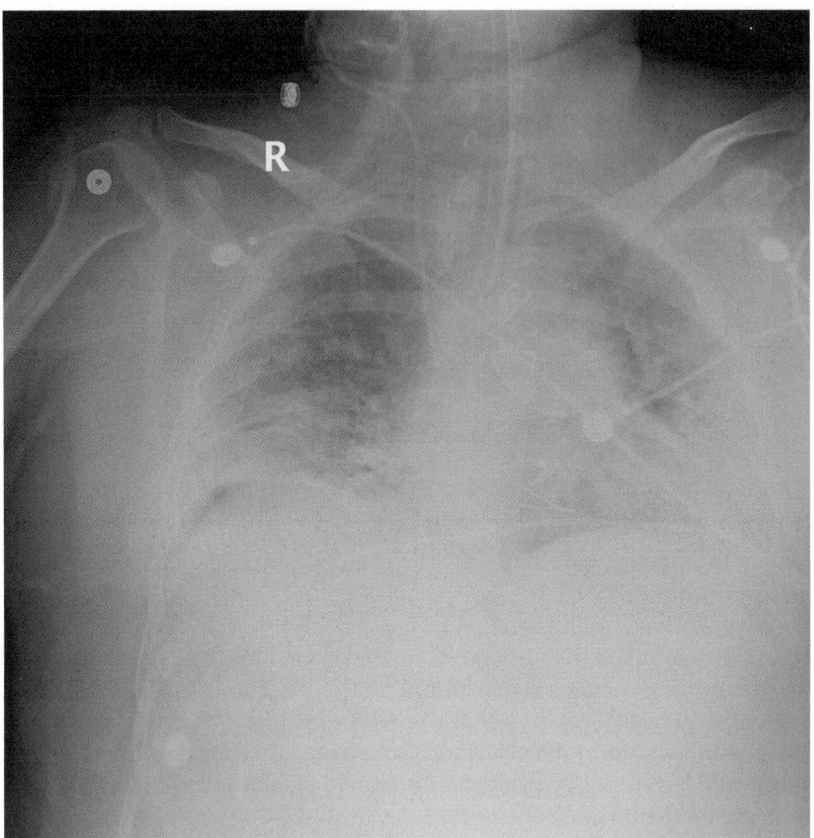

Figure 20.1 Chest x-ray demonstrating bilateral infiltrates typical of ALI/ARDS.

syndrome (ALI/ARDS) is an inflammatory condition of the lungs which can require a range of support from simple oxygen supplementation to advanced ventilatory support. It is defined as the acute onset of diffuse bilateral pulmonary infiltrates by chest radiograph as seen in Figure 20.1; a $PaO_2/FiO_2 < 300$ for ALI and < 200 for ARDS; and a pulmonary artery wedge pressure < 18 mm/Hg or no clinical evidence of fluid overload (Figure 20.1).

The causative factors can be divided into those associated with direct injury to the lung (e.g., aspiration, pneumonia, pulmonary contusion, fat emboli, and smoke or toxic gas inhalation) and those that cause indirect lung injury by inciting a systemic inflammatory response (e.g., sepsis, traumatic shock, pancreatitis, cardiopulmonary bypass, and blood transfusions). In the acute phase, leakage of edema into the lung and inflammatory cellular infiltrates causes ventilation–perfusion mismatch, which clinically manifests as hypoxemia. After the acute phase, some patients progress into a fibroproliferative phase, during which chronic inflammation and fibrosis take place, requiring prolonged ventilator support.

Chronic ventilator dependence

Prolonged mechanical ventilation is defined as ventilator dependence for greater than 21 days for at least 6 hours per day. Unlike acute respiratory insufficiency, chronic respiratory failure is often secondary to true pulmonary pathology or neuromuscular disease. These patients often require tracheostomy in an effort to increase the level of comfort, provide better oral care, reduce rates of pneumonia, and decrease dead space ventilation. Of the primary pulmonary disorders requiring prolonged mechanical ventilation, chronic obstructive pulmonary disease (COPD) is the most common. Obstructive or restrictive diseases manifest primarily as a ventilatory defect, with hypercapnea the end result. Oxygenation may also be affected due to perfusion defect. Decline in respiratory muscle function cannot compensate for the progressive increase in inspiratory volumes and overdistention that is classic with COPD, leading to worsening ventilator dependence.

Nutrition assessment

A comprehensive nutrition evaluation for patients with respiratory diseases should take into consideration the primary cause of pulmonary failure, as well as other associated co-morbidities. Establishing baseline deficits in patients with pulmonary failure is the first step in assessment. Standard physical exam and history should be performed, in addition to anthropometric measures. Fat-free mass index (FFMI) is considered as an alternative to BMI and a perhaps better indicator of nutrition in the critically ill population. Low fat-free mass index is positively correlated with airway obstruction, lung hyperinflation, and inspiratory load.

Estimating caloric needs will depend on the patient's illness acuity and trajectory. Greater variation in energy expenditure will occur during the early stages of illness, before a steady state has been achieved. The greater the degree of illness, the more susceptible the patient is to inaccuracies in estimation. Predictive equations are often used when deciding on the amount of target substrate. Although the REE is based on lean body mass, several factors influence the metabolic demand. Ventilated patients typically have many if not most of these factors, including infection, recent surgery, trauma, systemic inflammation, anasarca, and obesity. Conversion factors are used in some equations to account for these, but inaccuracies still exist when compared to indirect calorimetry measurements.

Indirect calorimetry

Indirect calorimetry (IC) is considered the gold standard for estimating resting energy expenditure (REE). This is particularly helpful in the acutely ill population and ventilated patients. Indirect calorimetry measures oxygen consumption (VO_2) and carbon dioxide excretion (VCO_2) as a representation of fuel combustion in the body. The two values are then used to calculate REE using the Weir equation. In the ventilated patient, IC may have technical limitations, and should not be used with elevated FiO_2 or PEEP levels or when an air leak in the circuit is present.

Indirect calorimetry may also be used to calculate the respiratory quotient (RQ). This is calculated as a ratio of carbon dioxide excretion to oxygen consumption and has previously been used to estimate carbohydrate vs lipid utilization. Although the RQ is tempting to use as a tool for adjusting substrate use, it should be employed with caution. The RQ value can be affected by other factors such as stress and hypermetabolism and may not accurately reflect individual substrate use. In more critically ill patients, it has been suggested that the RQ be used simply to validate the data provided by IC, i.e., if the value returned is not within a normal range, the REE calculated by IC is suspect. The RQ may also be helpful to determine overfeeding by any means.

One of the key therapeutic strategies for ventilated patients is limiting tidal volumes to prevent further inflammation and barotrauma. In doing so, the arterial CO_2 is allowed to rise until the pH reaches a set point before intervention is made to decrease alveolar CO_2 – what is known as permissive hypercapnea. For this reason, the minute ventilation for some patients with pulmonary failure, from ALI/ARDS and COPD in particular, cannot be manipulated as easily as other patients on mechanical ventilation. With this CO_2 release mechanism limited, it is even more imperative to tightly regulate the amount of CO_2 produced.

Overfeeding and CO_2 production

Overfeeding can lead to increased lipogenesis, increased glucose levels, and hepatic dysfunction. The type and amount of substrate delivered via nutritional support can also impact CO_2 production, making ventilator weaning difficult. Those patients most affected by overfeeding are typical of the ICU population: hyper-metabolic, nutritionally depleted, stressed, and those unable to eliminate CO_2. Patients with prolonged mechanical ventilator support can also suffer from overfeeding.

Carbohydrates have been implicated more often than simply excess calories in hypercapnea associated with overfeeding. Previous studies demonstrated that limiting carbohydrate administration resulted in reduced CO_2 elaboration, reduced the RQ, and improved respiratory outcomes, leading to a promotion of high-lipid "pulmonary formulas." A recent trial by Talpers et al. helped clarify this issue. When isocaloric diets were administered with varying concentrations of carbohydrate, CO_2 production was unchanged. With increasing caloric loads at a steady state carbohydrate concentration (60%), the CO_2 increased significantly. This and other studies confirmed that caloric overfeeding, not excess carbohydrate ratio, is the culprit in excess CO_2 production and failed ventilator weaning.

Enteral nutrition support

The merits of enteral nutrition for pulmonary failure patients are well established, particularly for preservation of gut mucosa and improved immunological function. Enteral provision is considered the route of choice for patients on the ventilator due to significantly reduced cost and rates of infection. Stimulation of gut-associated lymphoid tissue (GALT) by enteral nutrition has been reported to increase immunoglobulin A, which is protective against airway infections. Enteral provision should always be given in the setting of a functional gut and should be commenced as soon as resuscitation is complete. Further details of basic enteral nutritional support for mechanically ventilated critically ill patients has been summarily described in the society guidelines and the reader is re-directed there for further review.

Enteral nutrition delivery

Administering enteral nutrition in the ventilated patient requires a degree of dedication by the practitioner. Despite the numerous protective benefits of enteral nutrition, one of the greatest concerns in patients with pulmonary failure is its potential causality with aspiration and ventilator-associated pneumonia (VAP). Similarly, patients may suffer from aspiration pneumonitis, a condition in which gastric contents are aspirated into the respiratory tract, causing a chemical inflammatory reaction without secondary infection. Both conditions are devastating to mechanically ventilated patients.

Effective VAP prevention strategies target modifiable risk factors for colonization and aspiration, including elevation of the head of the bed to 30–45°, subglottic secretion draining, oral care with chlorhexidine, and minimizing the duration of mechanical ventilation. Reduction of gastroesophageal reflux has been demonstrated clinically with more distally placed tube feeds. Physiologically, feeding into the duodenum results in the same amount of gastroesophageal reflux as feeding into the stomach, therefore, tube placement into the jejunum is preferred. This may require endoscopy resources which are often limited; however, blind placement of a nasoenteric tube can often be successfully achieved as demonstrated in Figure 20.2. When gastric feeding must be utilized, strict adherence to aspiration precautions should be followed. Prokinetic agents are often used with enteral nutrition to promote gut motility. Metoclopramide and erythromycin are the most frequently used, although these may have less effect over time. Newer agents require further evaluation in the critically ill population.

Parenteral nutrition support

Patients with acute pulmonary failure often have other significant morbidities, of which shock, non-functional gut, and peritonitis can preclude appropriate enteral therapy. As noted in the ACCEPT study, survival benefits ensue when larger amounts of nutrient are delivered more consistently. The ESPEN guidelines for nutritional support endorse initiating supplemental PN at day 4 if 60% of EN goals are not met within 3 days. Although supplemental PN may be helpful in reducing the cumulative caloric deficit, this concept requires further clarification regarding composition, timing, and amount before advocating its use in pulmonary failure and critical care.

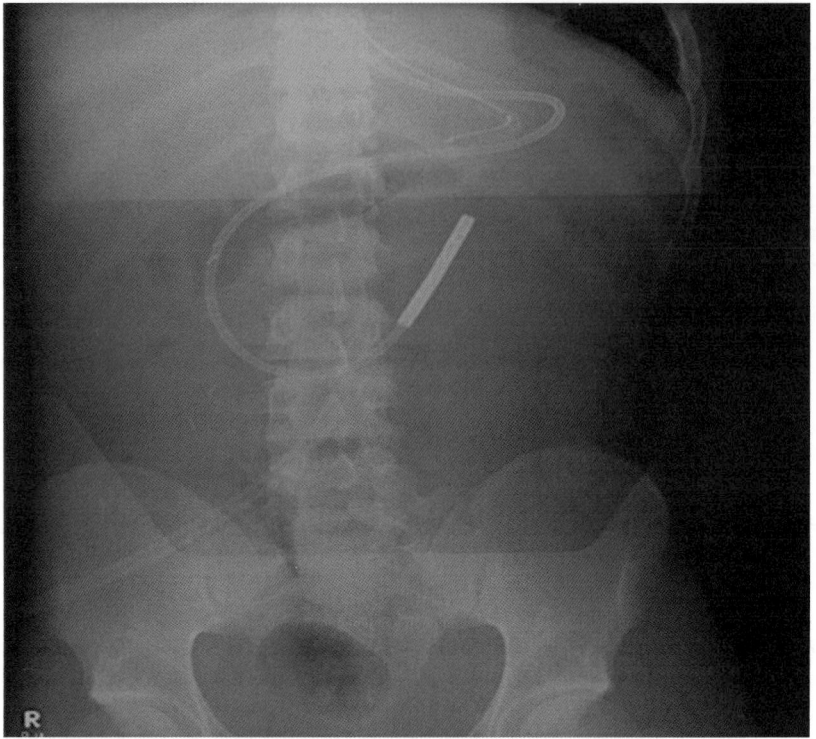

Figure 20.2 Abdominal x-ray demonstrating placement of nasoenteric feeding tube with the tip at the duodenal/jejuna junction.

Immunonutrition for respiratory diseases

Immunonutrition is the concept of providing nutritional substrate for the purpose of modulating immune function. Various substances have been investigated for this purpose, with the effect of reducing inflammation, enhancing healing, reducing rates of infection, and decreasing pulmonary morbidity as reflected by time required for mechanical ventilation. Agents investigated for these purposes include pre-biotics, probiotics, arginine, glutamine, antioxidants, and nucleic acids. Provision of omega-3 fatty acids for immune modulatory function has come under special scrutiny, and will therefore be examined more closely.

Omega-3 (n-3) fatty acids

Omega-3 fatty acids (n-3) consist of docosahexaenoic acid (DHA) and eicosapentaenoic acid (EPA) which are found predominantly in fish oils, as well as α-linolenic acid found in walnut and flax seed oils. These polyunsaturated fatty acids are metabolized to 3-series prostaglandins and 5-series leukotrienes, substances which reduce inflammation and eicosanoid production. Omega-6 fatty acids (n-6) and omega-9 fatty acids (n-9) are found predominantly in animal fat and consist of linolenic, dihomo-γ-linolenic acid, and arachidonic acid. Via a common enzyme pathway, n-6s are metabolized to 2-series prostaglandins, thromboxanes, and 4-series leukotrienes. These substances are pro-inflammatory in nature, influencing cytokine production, platelet aggregation, vasodilation, and vascular permeability. As an intermediate in the n-6 pathway, γ-linolenic acid (GLA) causes an increase in arachidonic acid levels. When GLA is administered with EPA, however, the terminal enzyme is blocked, reducing the resultant arachidonic acid production. This combination also leads to increased production of prostaglandin E_1, a potent pulmonary vasodilator.

As a primary inflammatory disorder, ALI/ARDS lends itself well to potential modulation by immunonutrition. A landmark paper published by Gadek et al. in 1999 utilized a commercial formulation of EPA, DHA, borage oil (containing GLA), and antioxidants for patients with ARDS. This study reported improved oxygenation and decreased ICU length of stay for patients receiving continuous infusion of the n-3-based formula versus a standard commercial pulmonary formula. Subsequent randomized controlled trials utilizing the same high n-3 ratio formula were published which likewise demonstrated improved pulmonary physiology, decreased ICU length of stay, decreased new organ failures, and decreased mortality. These findings led to a grade A (highest) recommendation for use of n-3 fatty acids in patients with ARDS by the ASPEN/SCCM guidelines.

Despite the initial enthusiasm for this formula for treatment of ARDS, numerous questions were raised. Of primary concern, the control group in these studies received a formula with a higher n-6 to n-3 ratio, exaggerating the potential anti-inflammatory effect of the n-3 supplementation. Likewise, it is unknown which component of the formula was responsible for the improved outcomes: EPA, DHA, GLA, antioxidants, or a particular combination of each. Additionally, lung protective ventilation strategies, which decrease systemic inflammation, were not universally applied to all patients in these initial studies and could influence the effects of further anti-inflammatory agents.

Subsequent trials were designed to address these questions. The investigators in a multi-center study randomized ALI/ARDS patients to receive either an n-3/GLA/antioxidant supplement or an isocaloric control supplement. The supplement was given enterally as a bolus twice daily independently of provision of EN by protocol. Despite an 8-fold increase in plasma EPA levels, patients who received the n-3 supplements failed to demonstrate any improvement in pulmonary physiology or clinical outcomes such as ventilator-free days, ICU-free days, organ failures or mortality.

An additional randomized controlled trial was completed during this same time period utilizing DHA and EPA supplements alone for patients with ALI/ARDS. This trial compared the n-3 supplements with saline placebo in a bolus fashion. No sources of GLA or antioxidants were administered. Additional enteral or parenteral nutrition provided was at the discretion of the clinician. This study likewise achieved significant serum levels of EPA; however, no differences in clinical out-comes were achieved. Additionally, serum and lung biomarkers of inflammation were unchanged in the study group.

Discordance among the initial and later trials requires further elucidation by larger trials. Questions about n-3 supplementation remain regarding timing and route of administration, duration of use, and optimal dose. Likewise, the specific effects of each component of the n-3 based formula need to be identified.

Summary points

- Pulmonary failure is an ongoing source of morbidity and mortality for critically ill patients.
- Estimating caloric requirements can be difficult due to co-morbidities and secondary diagnoses common to this population, and should be refined frequently to avoid overfeeding.
- Enteral feeding is preferred, with appropriate aspiration precautions vigilantly applied.
- Lipids should be provided to reduce carbohydrate load, and are increasingly used as immunonutrition.
- Supplementation with parenteral nutrition may be necessary in the early phases, but is also controversial and should be avoided long-term.
- Careful design of a nutrition plan, with frequent reassessment, is paramount to preventing further malnutrition and aiding with liberation from mechanical ventilation.

Further reading

Baker JP, Detsky AS, Stewart S, et al. Randomized trial of total parenteral nutrition in critically ill patients: metabolic effects of varying glucose-lipid ratios as the energy source. Gastroenterology 1984;87(1):53–59.

Blot S, Rello J, Vogelaers D. What is new in the prevention of ventilator-associated pneumonia? Curr Opin Pulm Med 2011;17(3):155–159.

Budweiser S, Meyer K, Jörres RA, et al. Nutritional depletion and its relationship to respiratory impairment in patients with chronic respiratory failure due to COPD or restrictive thoracic diseases. Eur J Clin Nutr 2008;62(3):436–443.

Gadek JE, DeMichele SJ, Karlstad MD, et al. Effect of enteral feeding with eicosapenta-enoic acid, gamma-linolenic acid, and antioxidants in patients with acute respiratory distress syndrome. Enteral Nutrition in ARDS Study Group. Crit Care Med 1999;27 (8):1409–1420.

Kreymann KG, Berger MM, Deutz NEP, et al. ESPEN Guidelines on Enteral Nutrition: Intensive care. Clin Nutr 2006;25(2):210–223.

Martin CM, Doig GS, Heyland DK, Morrison T, Sibbald WJ. Multicentre, cluster-randomized clinical trial of algorithms for critical-care enteral and parenteral therapy (ACCEPT). CMAJ 2004;170(2):197–204.

McClave SA, Martindale RG, Vanek VW, et al. Guidelines for the Provision and Assessment of Nutrition Support Therapy in the Adult Critically Ill Patient: Society of Critical Care Medicine (SCCM) and American Society for Parenteral and Enteral Nutrition (A.S.P.E.N.). J Parenter Enteral Nutr 2009;33(3):277–316.

Pontes-Arruda A, Aragão AMA, Albuquerque JD. Effects of enteral feeding with eicosapentaenoic acid, gamma-linolenic acid, and antioxidants in mechanically ventilated patients with severe sepsis and septic shock. Crit Care Med 2006;34(9):2325–2333.

Rice TW, Wheeler AP, Thompson BT, et al. Enteral omega-3 fatty acid, gamma-linolenic acid, and antioxidant supplementation in acute lung injury. JAMA 2011;306(14):1574–1581.

Singer P, Theilla M, Fisher H, et al. Benefit of an enteral diet enriched with eicosapentaenoic acid and gamma-linolenic acid in ventilated patients with acute lung injury. Crit Care Med 2006;34(4):1033–1038.

Stapleton RD, Martin TR, Weiss NS, et al. A phase II randomized placebo-controlled trial of omega-3 fatty acids for the treatment of acute lung injury. Crit Care Med 2011;39(7):1655–1662.

Talpers SS, Romberger DJ, Bunce SB, Pingleton SK. Nutritionally associated increased carbon dioxide production. Excess total calories vs high proportion of carbohydrate calories. Chest 1992;102(2):551–555.

Wheeler AP, Bernard GR. Acute lung injury and the acute respiratory distress syndrome: a clinical review. Lancet 2007;369(9572):1553–1564.

21

Nutritional support of critically ill organ transplantation patients

Andrew J. Kerwin and Michael S. Nussbaum

Introduction

Organ transplantation has become a life-saving procedure for patients with end stage kidney, liver, lung, and heart disease. However, these patients are typically debilitated and malnourished prior to undergoing transplantation. The surgical literature is replete with studies documenting the increased morbidity and mortality following non-transplant surgery on malnourished patients. In an effort to achieve the best outcomes following organ transplantation transplant surgeons have also tried to study the effects of malnutrition on outcomes following organ transplantation. They have looked at the relationship of malnutrition to infectious complications, graft function, hospital length of stay, intensive care unit length of stay, and mortality.

Etiology of malnutrition

The etiology of malnutrition in patients with end stage disease is complex and multifactorial. In patients with renal failure the loss of kidney function results in acidosis that induces protein catabolism and alters amino acid uptake thus negatively affecting nitrogen balance. There is also a negative effect on albumin synthesis and albumin concentration. The hormonal milieu is deranged as well. In addition, nutritional intake can be poor due to anorexia, hospitalization, gastroparesis, nausea, vomiting, and poor tasting specialized diets among other things.

Similarly, the etiology of malnutrition in liver disease is also multifactorial (Figure 21.1). Patients with liver disease also have decreased caloric intake for similar reasons to those in patients with renal failure. Autonomic dysfunction of liver disease leads to gastroparesis, a delay in small bowel motility, and ultimately a delay in gastrointestinal transit. When this is combined with ascites the result is nausea and early satiety. Ascites is also responsible for increased protein loss which in combination with altered protein metabolism results in overall protein loss.

Nutrition in Critical Care, ed. Peter Faber and Mario Siervo. Published by Cambridge University Press. © Cambridge University Press 2014.

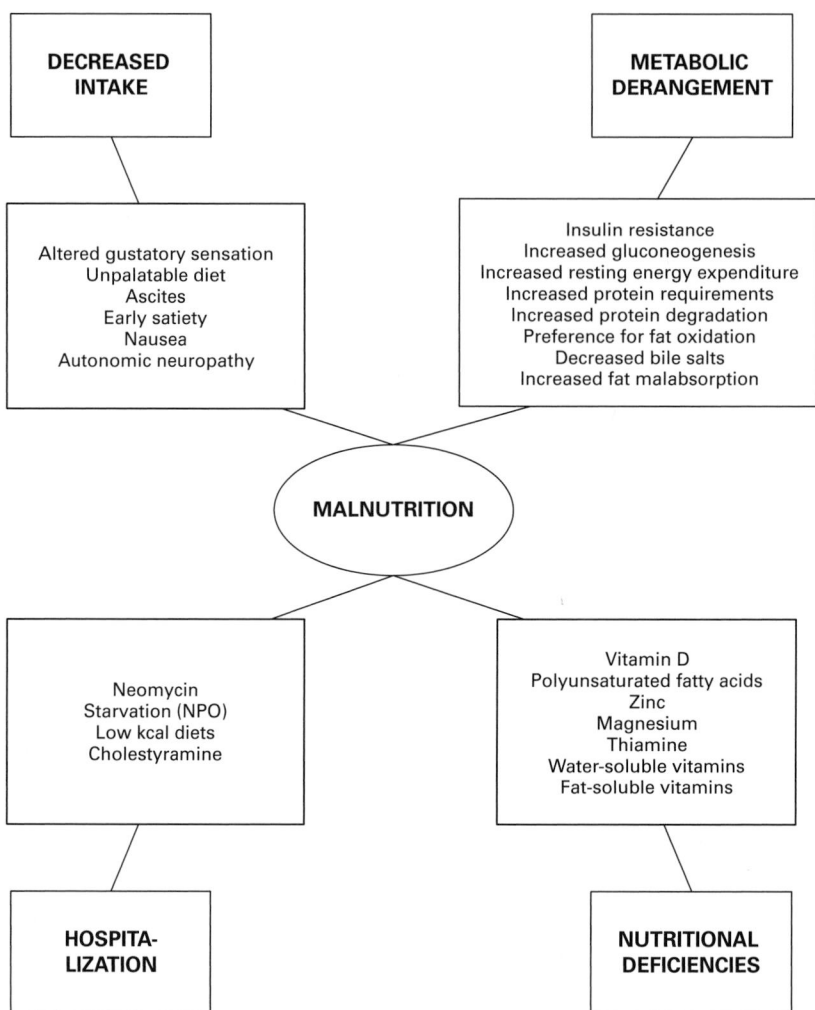

Figure 21.1 Multiple contributing etiologies of malnutrition in patients with liver disease.

The derangements in the physiology of metabolism that occur in patients with liver failure are complex and further add to malnutrition. The disease state is characterized as a hyper-metabolic state with glucose intolerance. The glucose intolerance is a key abnormality that can result in diabetes mellitus. The etiology of the hyper-metabolic state is unclear but may be related to increased sympathetic nervous system activity. In liver disease there is a decrease in glycogen stores with a resultant increase in gluconeogenesis that results in a shift from carbohydrate metabolism to a preference for fat metabolism.

There are multiple vitamin and micronutrient deficiencies that accompany liver disease. Deficiencies in both the water-soluble and fat-soluble vitamins have been described. Both magnesium and zinc deficiencies have been described as well. However, it remains controversial as to whether or not zinc supplementation is beneficial.

Malnutrition in patients with end stage cardiac disease is also common. Similarly, the etiology is multifactorial as well. Cardiac cachexia is a well known problem in patients with heart failure. In addition, heart failure is a hyper-metabolic state with a tendency towards decreased nutritional intake due to things such as dyspnea, intestinal edema, liver congestion, and hospitalizations. Cardiac ischemia results in an alteration of glucose utilization and a shift to anaerobic glycolysis. There are also deficiencies of thiamine, selenium, L-carnitine, coenzyme Q10, the B vitamins, and vitamins C, D, and E which contribute to the develop-ment of malnutrition in cardiac failure in addition to negatively affecting cardiac function.

Nutritional assessment

In order to achieve optimal results following transplantation it is vital for surgeons to get an accurate and reliable assessment of the nutritional status in the pre-operative planning stages. While this may seem to be an easy assessment, it actually turns out to be rather challenging. For example, despite the fact that malnutrition is nearly ubiquitous in liver disease, determining an accurate assess-ment of a patient's nutritional status is difficult due to such things as ascites, peripheral edema, and protein wasting. These aspects of liver disease make tradi-tional assessment tools inaccurate and leave us to search for a "gold standard" assessment tool.

There are multitudes of ways to assess nutritional status in potential transplant patients including detailed history and physical exam, biochemical measurements, measured indices, and sophisticated bioelectrical impedance analysis. The initial assessment of the potential transplant patient should begin with a careful history to elucidate such things as nausea, vomiting, diarrhea, early satiety, changes in taste, weight loss, specialized diets and supplements, and recent dietary intake. A complete physical examination should look for signs of peripheral edema, ascites, palmar erythema, spider angiomas, loss of subcutaneous fat, and muscle wasting.

Biochemical tests of nutritional status include pre-albumin, transferrin, retinol binding protein, urine nitrogen balance, and creatinine-height index. Given the catabolic nature of liver disease and the associated protein turnover these measure-ments have not been shown to be accurate. The most important measure of nutritional status in this patient population is the serum albumin level.

Objective measurements have been suggested as a more reliable and accurate way to assess nutritional status. BMI is one such measure although its accuracy has been questioned depending on the presence of peripheral edema or ascites. Researchers have evaluated the BMI in relation to the presence of ascites and have been able to identify optimal BMI levels in patients with ascites in order to prevent post-operative complications.

Anthropometric measures such as mid-arm muscle circumference and triceps skin fold thickness have also been used as part of a nutritional assessment. When compared to a clinical assessment based on history and physical examination, it was found that in 23% of patients the clinical assessment differed from the anthropometric measures. The clinical assessment underestimated the nutritional abnormalities. Based on this the authors suggested that anthropometric measures be incorporated into the nutritional assessment of patients with liver disease. Unfortunately, these measures have been called into question over concerns of inter-rater reliability and the reliability in patients with ascites.

Subjective global assessment (SGA) is a clinical tool first described over two decades ago and has been used to assess nutritional status in liver disease as well as other disease states. It combines a thorough history and physical looking for signs of muscle wasting and loss of subcutaneous fat in order to classify patients as well nourished, moderately, or severely malnourished. While this tool seems simple it has been criticized because of concerns of accuracy. However, Duerksen has shown that the SGA can be taught to medical students and they were able to reliably classify patients as either moderately or severely malnourished.

Nutritional therapy

Since it appears that malnutrition is nearly universal in patients with end stage renal, pulmonary, cardiac, and liver disease, nutritional support is essential. The evidence is clear that malnutrition is linked to worse outcomes in surgical patients undergoing major procedures and it appears to be true for patients undergoing organ transplantation. Although there is some debate about method of nutrition delivery there is consensus that enteral nutrition is the optimal route of delivery of nutrition for all patients who are not able to maintain adequate oral intake. It is well accepted that the use of enteral nutrition is less costly and associated with fewer complications and decreased hospital length of stay as compared to parenteral nutrition. Published guidelines from the Society of Critical Care Medicine (SCCM), the ASPEN, and also the European Society for Clinical Nutrition and Metabolism (ESPEN) provide us with guidance for delivery of nutrition to these critically ill patients.

Given that malnutrition is almost universal in this patient population, potential transplant patients should be assessed for signs of malnutrition using the methods described above once they are placed on the transplant waiting list. Multiple studies have shown that patients with low BMI pre-transplant will have greater morbidity and mortality in the post-operative period than those patients who have a normal BMI. Patients should try to meet their caloric needs with their oral intake but if they are not able to do so then they should use oral supplements. Their goal should be to eat enough so as to maintain a normal BMI. Incorporating a multi-disciplinary nutrition support team with a dietician and a nutritional intervention program is essential in the pre-operative phase for patients that are placed on the transplant list. Patients awaiting liver transplantation should target a caloric goal of 35–40 kcal/kg body weight/day with a protein intake goal of 1.2–1.5 g/kg body weight/day. It was previously believed that patients with liver disease should have their protein intake limited. However this is no longer believed to be true. Limiting the protein intake in patients with liver failure has been associated with increased mortality.

Another area of great debate for patients with liver failure has been the use of branched-chain amino acid (BCAA – leucine, isoleucine, and valine) enhanced supplements. The BCAA do not require the liver for metabolism and are thus preferentially used by the failing liver, while aromatic amino acids (AAA – phenyl-alanine, tryptophan, and tyrosine) are not metabolized effectively in liver failure and accumulate. This altered protein metabolism leads to a reduction in the BCAA and an increase in the circulating levels of the AAA. This imbalance between the AAA and the BCAA may play a role in the hepatic encephalopathy. While this has been vigorously debated it appears that supplementation with BCAA produces modest improvement in hepatic encephalopathy at best and no improvement in mortality.

Even though enteral nutrition is the preferred route of nutritional supplementation in patients with end stage disease who are not able to maintain adequate oral intake, there are still times when parenteral nutrition must be used as an alternative route. For patients who are moderately or severely malnourished and cannot achieve adequate caloric intake either orally or through enteral feedings, parenteral nutrition should be initiated. It is also appropriate to commence parenteral nutrition in patients fasting for more than 72 hours. Given the low glycogen stores in patients with liver disease it is important to provide a glucose infusion in these patients if they are not able to take oral nutrients or enteral nutrition for more than 12 hours. The glucose infusion should be adjusted to supply 2–3 g/kg body weight/day of glucose.

If full parenteral nutrition is required the energy goal should be $1.3 \times$ the REE. Carbohydrates should comprise 50–60% of the total non-protein energy requirements while lipids should make up the remaining 40–50%. Just as when using enteral nutrition, parenteral nutrition should provide 1.2–1.5 g amino acids/kg body weight/day. For patients with compensated cirrhosis 1.2 g amino acids/kg body weight/day is sufficient but for those with decompensated cirrhosis the protein infusion should be increased to provide 1.5 g/kg body weight/day.

There are some different considerations for patients who present with ALF although the data in this area is limited. If these patients are not likely to resume normal oral intake within 5–7 days parenteral nutrition should be initiated. Amino acids should be administered in acute or subacute liver failure but are not mandatory in hyper-acute liver failure. The goal for these patients is 0.8–1.2 g amino acids/kg body weight/day.

Patients in the immediate post-transplant period should be approached in a similar manner as other post-surgical patients in terms of their nutritional requirements. Guidelines for nutritional support of the critically ill post-surgical patient have been compiled and are well known. Many transplant patients will be able to resume oral intake shortly after their transplant but if they are unable to resume normal oral intake promptly then enteral nutrition should begin as early as 12 hours post-transplant. Obtaining feeding access is especially easy in liver transplant patients who can have a feeding jejunostomy tube inserted at the time of their transplant. Resuming enteral nutrition within 12 hours of transplant has been shown to reduce post-operative viral infections and produce better nitrogen retention. Ensuring adequate nutritional intake and correction of vitamin and micronutrient deficiencies *may* help reduce peri-operative morbidity and mortality following liver transplantation.

The guidelines for suggested caloric and protein intake in the immediate post-operative period are as stated above. Again, the enteral route is preferred compared with the parenteral route. The caloric target for liver transplant patients is 35–40 kcal/kg body weight/day with a protein intake target of 1.2–1.5 g/kg body weight/day. Post-kidney transplant and post-lung transplant patients have a suggested caloric goal of 30–35 kcal/kg body weight/day and protein goal of 1.3–1.5 g/kg body weight/day.

There are several areas of new research in the nutrition support of organ transplant patients. Some recent evidence suggests that use of immune-modulating diets and probiotic agents in the immediate post liver transplant patient may help reduce infections while not interfering with the necessary immuno-suppression required. Researchers have also begun to examine the utility of BCAA supplementation in the peri-operative period and its relationship to outcome following liver transplantation. Additionally, the use of vitamin D supplementation is being analyzed to determine the impact on post-transplant infection, rejection, and graft survival. These exciting areas of research will certainly require further investigation to determine if indeed there is a benefit to utilizing these therapies.

Conclusions

Patients with end stage disease requiring organ transplantation are complex and present physicians with difficult challenges. Malnutrition is nearly universal and needs to be addressed as part of the pre-operative preparation. A thorough nutritional assessment is important to uncover signs of malnutrition and treat it prior to undergoing a transplant. A subjective global assessment may be the best technique but there is no consensus as to which technique is the gold standard for making such an assessment. For patients who cannot achieve adequate oral intake, enteral nutrition via a nasogastric tube is the preferred route of delivery with a goal of 35–40 kcal/kg body weight/day and 1.2–1.5 g protein/kg body weight/day following liver transplant and 30–35 kcal/kg body weight/day and protein goal of 1.3–1.5 g/kg body weight/day following kidney or lung transplant. These same goals should be targeted for liver transplant patients whether in the pre- or post-operative period.

Summary points

- Patients awaiting transplant surgery are universally malnourished.
- Nutritional assessment involves clinical examination and biochemical tests. Patients should be nutritionally optimized prior to transplant surgery.

- Care is advised in applying prevalent clinical assessment tools in this group of patients. The Subjective Global Assessment tool is relatively reliable and easy to use.
- Patients in liver failure may benefit from receiving branched-chain amino acids as compared with aromatic amino acids.
- Total calorie intake should be 30–35 kcal/kg body weight/day in most transplant patients.

Further reading

Braga M, Ljungqvist O, Soeters P, et al. ESPEN Guidelines on Parenteral Nutrition: Surgery. Clin Nutr 2009;28:378–386.

Detsky AS, McLaughlin JR, Baker JP, et al. What is subjective global assessment of nutritional status? J Parenter Enteral Nutr 1987;11(1):8–13.

Kerwin AJ, Nussbaum MS. Adjuvant nutrition management of patients with liver failure including transplantation. Surg Clin North Am 2011;565–578.

Martindale RG, McClave SA, Vanek VW, et al. Guidelines for the provision and assessment of nutrition support therapy in the adult critically ill patient: Society of Critical Care Medicine and American Society for Parenteral and Enteral Nutrition. Crit Care Med 2009;37(5):1–30.

Martins C, Pecoits-Filho R, Riella MC. Nutrition for the post-renal transplant recipients. Transplant Proc 2004;36:1650–1654.

Molnar MZ, Kvesdy CP, Bunnapradist S, et al. Associations of pretransplant serum albumin with post-transplant outcomes in kidney transplant recipients. Am J Transplant 2011;11:1006–1015.

Plauth M, Cabre E, Riggio O, et al. ESPEN Guidelines on Enteral Nutrition: Liver disease. Clin Nutr 2006;25:285–294.

Sarma S, Gheorghiade M. Nutritional assessment and support of the patient with acute heart failure. Curr Opin Crit Care 2010;16:413–418.

Stein EM, Shane E. Vitamin D in organ transplantation. Osteoporos Int 2011;22:2107–2018.

Weimann A, Braga M, Harsanyi L, et al. ESPEN Guidelines on Enteral Nutrition: Surgery including organ transplantation. Clin Nutr 2006;25:224–244.

22

Nutritional management of anorexia in critical care

Maria Gabriella Gentile

Introduction

Anorexia nervosa (AN) exhibits one of the highest mortalities of any psychiatric condition and a relevant fraction of it comes from undernutrition. Guidelines suggest that an AN patient weighing less than 70% of ideal body weight or with BMI lower than 15 kg/m^2 should be considered to be affected by severe anorexia nervosa and warrant admission for medical stabilization and management of the complications of severe malnutrition.

Severe and protracted undernutrition nearly always leads to marked changes in body spaces (e.g., intra-extracellular water), and in body masses (e.g., phosphate, potassium, magnesium overall, and compartmental stores). Detailed clinical findings are: hemodynamic instability, severe volume derangement (depletion or overhydration), bradycardia (≤ 45–50 beats per minute), bone marrow depression, severe electrolyte disturbances including metabolic alkalosis, hypoglycemia, hypothermia from reduced basal metabolic rate, and euthyroid sick syndrome. These changes set the body at risk of refeeding syndrome, i.e., the disturbances caused by a too rapid/ unbalanced refeeding which the referred to deranged bodily system is unable to stand.

There are unique aspects of AN patients: awareness of illness (and/or its consequences) is scarce or none; even in life-threatening situations these patients do not want to be cured and are vigorously opposed to treatment. They can mask their true weight by drinking water or bearing weights or other objects; they try to purge even as inpatients; food and drugs may be hidden or eliminated; and intravenous drip discontinued (Table 22.1).

Aims of treatment

The treatment goals for AN include:
• Preventing and/or curing morbidity and mortality by restoring body weight, correcting biological and psychological sequelae of malnutrition, avoiding refeeding syndrome.

Nutrition in Critical Care, ed. Peter Faber and Mario Siervo. Published by Cambridge University Press. © Cambridge University Press 2014.

Table 22.1 Severe anorexia nervosa: principal signs and symptoms

Medical complications
–   Cardiovascular: low blood pressure, bradycardia, decreased voltage and prolonged QTc
–   Metabolic: metabolism slowing, hypoglycemia, hypothermia, euthyroid sick syndrome, bone marrow depression
–   Abnormal liver function
–   Abnormalities in brain functions
Psychological signs
–   Refusal to acknowledge the gravity of illness
–   Low self-esteem
–   Overvaluations of appearance
–   Obsessive-compulsive behavior
–   Depression-anxiety
–   Insomnia-restlessness
Behavioral symptoms
–   Refusal of medical treatments (drugs, nutrition, bed rest)
–   Obsession with calories, fat grams
–   Compulsive exercising
–   Falsify their body weight
–   Use of purging behavior (vomiting/ purging)

● Correcting dysfunctional behaviors and thinking.
● Treating depression and obsessive thinking.
● Restoring autonomy and preventing relapse and disablement.
● Supporting family or partner.

Category A evidence-based treatment of AN is still lacking, but international guidelines and society position papers agree on the fact that the best treatment should involve a multi-disciplinary process performed by a team of medical, nutritional, mental health, and nursing professionals trained on the management of eating disorders.

Assessment of clinical and nutritional status

A complete history should be taken to determine illness duration and medical history, and a complete evaluation of primary clinical variables such as heart rate, ECG, and systolic and diastolic blood pressure should be made.

Circulatory volume should be evaluated with care because these patients may be dehydrated or overhydrated and suffer from poor myocardial contractility. Undernutrition may cause relevant electrocardiographic changes such as prolongation of QT interval with an increased risk of life-threatening arrhythmias, in particular torsade de pointes. Electrolyte disturbances which further increase the risk of serious arrhythmias and vitamin deficiencies are frequent. These aspects are crucially relevant during the refeeding, when electrolyte derangements can actually arise or be aggravated. Body weight and height are to be measured at the beginning of and during refeeding.

Body composition may be estimated by bioelectrical impedance analysis and dual X-ray absorptiometry (DXA). Resting energy expenditure should be evaluated by indirect calorimetry (IC).

Laboratory values

Hematological and biochemical assessment should include: anemia related test, glucose, liver and renal function, amylase, plasma electrolytes, phosphate, and magnesium. Glycemia, phosphate, magnesium, potassium, and sodium should be monitored daily and eventually corrected, if required.

Assessment of behaviors

Investigation and search for vomiting or purging, use of laxatives, diuretics, or other weight-regulating substances are mandatory. It is essential to remember that often these patients can deny any purging behavior and, therefore, clues should be searched for.

Nutritional and medical treatment

Refeeding of severely malnourished patients represents two very difficult and conflicting tasks: (1) avoid "refeeding syndrome" caused by too fast correction of malnutrition, (2) avoid "underfeeding syndrome" caused by a too cautious rate of refeeding. Caloric intake should be planned starting with indirect calorimetric measurements, because resting energy expenditure (REE) is the main component of daily expenditure particularly in severely and chronically malnourished patients; otherwise we should estimate energy needs taking into consideration that severely undernourished patients have an estimated energy need of 70–80% with respect to the Harris–Benedict formula. In a study on 33 AN patients affected by severe undernutrition (BMI 11.3 ± 0.7 kg/m^2) mean measured REE was 27.3 ± 4.4 kcal/kg/day, which means a negative difference versus REE estimated basal metabolic rate according to the Harris–Benedict formula of 29.5 ± 1.3%.

Although it has always been stressed how crucial nutritional rehabilitation is in these patients, there are only a few studies that report on artificial nutrition in AN patients. Both enteral and parenteral nutrition are used, but evidence-based guidelines on the issues is lacking. Since the international guidelines on the use of artificial nutrition state "if the gut works you must use it," we should choose enteral nutrition also for those AN patients who require life-saving artificial nutrition. Enteral feeding, like every other medical treatment, has to be closely monitored and regulated via an electronically operated pump. Nasogastric feeding is preferable because, compared with other methods, it has a lower risk of complications and is cost-efficient. In more compliant patients it is possible to use oral liquid supplements.

Table 22.2 Specific enteral nutrition protocol for anorexia nervosa patient

Formula	Calorie dense 1.7–2 kcal/mL
	Caloric distribution (% of kcal)
	– Protein 17%
	– Carbohydrate 43%
	– Fat 40%
Delivery site	
Route	Gastric
Access	Nasogastric
Method of administration	Pump–assisted
Rate of administration	Initial 20–30 mL/h
	Advance to goal of 40–60 mL/h or more if tolerated, for 24 h per day
Other indications	Flush the feeding tube with indicated amount of water every 6–8 h
Monitoring	Check gastric residual volume according to individual necessity
	Observe for abdominal distension
	Weigh daily

Oral feeding should never be stopped; the committed dietician team must develop and implement a personalized meal plan that suits the changing needs and ensures all major food groups. Enteral nutrition should begin as soon as possible, usually 1–3 hours after patient admission. To avoid fluid overload and to reduce gastric discomfort, high-caloric (1.7–2 kcal/mL), polymeric, lactose-free, gluten-free, high-nitrogen (17% of kcal intake), completely fluid-formula diets are commercially available (Table 22.2).

The flow rate should be kept constant for 24 hours using a pump, starting with an initial rate of 20–30 mL/hour and with progressive acceleration, if tolerated, up to 40–60 mL/hour. The goal is to obtain a weekly average weight gain of 0.5–1 kg, which means an excess of around 3500–7000 kcal a week. Prevention of hypoglycemia requires special care in patients suffering from extreme undernutrition. The combined use of continuous enteral nutrition and intravenous fluid containing 5–10% glucose (20–40 mL/hour) for 24 hours may prevent hypoglycemic episodes, which is virtually always possible because the liver lacks sufficient substrate to maintain the patient's serum glucose.

Vitamin and electrolyte supplementations

Thiamine and other B vitamins should be supplemented from the very beginning and should continue during refeeding days. The optimal amount of vitamin and micronutrient supplementations is unknown; doubling the daily recommended intake of vitamin and trace elements appears beneficial. Vitamin K should be

Table 22.3 Algorithm for treatment of extremely undernourished subjects with anorexia nervosa

---

1. Restore circulatory volume, monitor fluid balance, blood pressure, heart rate, ECG, if necessary cardiac monitoring
2. Take blood samples: electrolyte levels should be monitored especially at baseline and replaced as needed
3. Give oral/enteral thiamine and vitamin B two times daily
4. Start administration of intravenous fluid with 5–10% glucose (20–40 mL/hour)
5. Start slowly with enteral feeding or oral nutritional supplements
6. Start immediately with phosphate supplements oral/NG/or i.v. infusion
7. Start with potassium, magnesium supplements as soon as you have plasma levels
8. Monitor body temperature and correct hypothermia with blankets and appropriate clothes
9. Organize and monitor bed rest

IV, intravenous; NG, nasogastric.

prescribed according to blood values. In patients at risk of refeeding syndrome it is indicated to start phosphate oral supplements, such as KPhos and/or i.v. as NaPhos even before the complete serum electrolyte panel is available. The starting phosphate dose has to be evaluated in each patient according to the degree of undernutrition, and subsequently on the basis of the rate of rebuilding cells and organs. The amounts to be provided are highly variable and require strict, daily monitoring of serum phosphate. Phosphate supplementation can range from 10 to 40 mmol/day with an average of about 20 mmol/day. Potassium and magnesium supplements are usually required and may need daily adjustments according to blood levels.

Hydration and body weight modification

Body weight must be checked at least once a day. Body fluid deficits and/or losses should be carefully replaced according to circulatory and renal function. Oral intake of water should be carefully prescribed and monitored. Due to often excessive consumption of water AN patients are at risk of fluid overload. Daily requirements are usually 25–30 mL/kg/day (Table 22.3).

Discussion

The crude mortality rate of AN patients in critical care is still high (about 10%), and prevention of refeeding syndrome is essential to reduce it. In order to ameliorate the effects of catabolic processes and prevent refeeding syndrome it is important to prescribe a caloric intake that is higher than estimated from measurements of REE.

The continuous monitoring of fluid intake is necessary to avoid refeeding edema and cardiac failure. Enteral nutrition with a high-calorie solution is usually well tolerated if treatment is enforced by an empathic team approach.

Enteral nutrition should be considered first; parenteral nutrition may produce an even higher risk of refeeding syndrome. Prevention and treatment of hypo-phosphatemia is key to dealing with these patients; generous and continuous phosphate supplementation is needed from the outset and throughout the refeeding period.

Psychiatrists can and should help in managing behavioral problems, such as sabotaging feeding and drugs therapy, and in the treatment of possible significant co-morbid psychopathology with psychotropic drugs. Establishing a good relationship with family members early on may prevent and/or reduce the necessity of instituting compulsory treatment, according to local legislation.

Summary points

- Anorexia nervosa exhibits one of the highest mortalities of any psychiatric condition and a relevant fraction of it comes from undernutrition.
- The best treatment for AN should involve a multi-disciplinary process performed by a team of medical, nutritional, mental health, and nursing professionals trained on the management of eating disorders.
- Enteral feeding should be closely monitored and the nasogastric route should be considered first.
- Caloric intake should be planned to obtain a weekly average weight gain of 0.5–1 kg, which means an excess of around 3500–7000 kcal a week.
- Refeeding of severely malnourished patients should aim to avoid "refeeding syndrome" while providing an adequate caloric intake to restore normal bodily functions.
- The optimal amount of vitamin and micronutrient supplementations is unknown; doubling the daily recommended intake of vitamin and trace elements appears beneficial.
- Prevention and treatment of hypophosphatemia is a key point of the nutritional support.

Further reading

American Psychiatric Association Work Group on Eating Disorders. Practice guideline for the treatment of patients with eating disorders. 2006.

Byrnes MC, Stangenes J. Refeeding in the ICU: an adult and pediatric problem. Curr Opin Clin Nutr Metab Care 2011;14:186–192.

Gaudiani JL, Sabel AL, Mascolo M, Mehler PS. Severe anorexia nervosa: outcomes from a Medical Stabilization Unit. Int J Eat Disord 2012;45:85–92.

Gentile MG, Manna GM, Ciceri R, Rodeschini E. Efficacy of inpatient treatment in severely malnourished anorexia nervosa patients. Eat Weight Disord 2008;13:191–197.

Gentile MG, Pastorelli P, Ciceri R, et al. Specialized refeeding treatment for anorexia nervosa patients suffering from extreme undernutrition. Clin Nutr 2010;29:627–632.

Kohn MR, Madden S, Clarke SD. Refeeding in anorexia nervosa: increased safety and efficiency through understanding the pathophysiology of protein calorie malnutrition. Curr Opin Pediatr 2011;23:390–394.

MARSIPAM Group. MARSIPAN: Management of Really Sick Patients with Anorexia Nervosa. London: Royal College of Psychiatrists and Royal College of Physicians; 2010.

Mehanna HM, Moledina J, Travis J. Refeeding syndrome: what it is, and how to prevent and treat it. BMJ 2008;336:1495–1498.

Sylvester CJ, Forman SF. Clinical practice guidelines for treating restrictive eating disorder patients during medical hospitalization. Curr Opin Pediatr 2008;20:390–397.

Vignaud M, Constantin J-M, Ruivard M, et al. Refeeding syndrome influences outcome of anorexia nervosa patients in intensive care unit: an observational study. Crit Care 2010;14:R172.

23

Nutritional support of critically ill obese patients

Dong Wook Kim and Caroline M. Apovian

Introduction

The World Health Organization (WHO) defines "overweight" as a BMI between 25 and 29.9 kg/m², and "obesity" as a BMI of 30 kg/m² or higher. Obesity has become a global epidemic weighing heavily on the healthcare system. There are more than 1.5 billion overweight adults of whom at least 500 million are obese worldwide. The rising obese population and accompanying obesity-related issues frequently pose challenges in ICUs. Approximately 25–30% of patients admitted to the ICU have a BMI > 30 kg/m² in the United States. Intensive care in obese patients is more challenging than in non-obese patients primarily due to obesity-induced physiological complications such as hyperglycemia, immobility, thromboembolic disease, impaired hepatic function, and a pre-existing inflammatory state. Moreover, the physical aspects of severe obesity frequently require the use of specialized equipment such as special beds, lifts, long instruments, etc. to provide appropriate care to obese patients. In addition, routine procedures such as insertion of central venous catheters or arterial lines can be risky in severely obese patients.

The effect of obesity on mortality in the ICU is a controversial topic. Several observational studies have shown obesity to have a protective effect in critically ill patients, and in these studies was associated with improved outcomes. This phenomenon has been dubbed the "obesity paradox." However, a recent prospective study showed a higher mortality in obese patients (average BMI 34 kg/m²) with a predominant abdominal fat distribution and it concluded that a high sagittal abdominal diameter is an independent risk factor in the ICU. A multi-center international observational study (355 ICUs in 33 countries) showed that a BMI >40 kg/m² is associated with prolonged mechanical ventilation in the ICU. Obesity does not protect against adverse nutritional states and acute malnutrition. Although obese patients may have a high energy reservoir due to their large fat mass, these fuels may not be utilized effectively due to metabolic derangements

Nutrition in Critical Care, ed. Peter Faber and Mario Siervo. Published by Cambridge University Press. © Cambridge University Press 2014.

such as insulin resistance, impaired glucose tolerance, and increased fatty acid mobilization. Altered fuel metabolism in obesity may actually predispose patients to a greater loss of lean body mass and nutritional stress, which can lead to sarcopenic obesity. Therefore, proper nutritional assessment and nutrition support are important elements in managing critically ill obese patients, which this chapter will review.

Estimating energy requirements

Currently, indirect calorimetry (IC) is one of the most accurate methods available to assess the energy requirements in critically ill patients, including the obese. There are many equations, which have been evaluated to estimate energy requirements. However, they all are associated with significant error, especially in the critically ill obese patients as they are typically derived from the non-obese and non-critically ill population. For example, using the equation from the 1997 ACCP guideline (25–30 kcal/kg/day of actual body weight) would overestimate the caloric needs of critically ill patients that are obese. Since adipose tissue is less metabolically active than fat-free mass, using actual body weight is likely to overestimate caloric needs. Multiple studies have attempted to validate the use of equations such as the Harris-Benedict or Mifflin–St Jeor calculations in obese patients and have shown conflicting results. Recently, the Society of Critical Care Medicine (SCCM) and American Society for Parenteral and Enternal Nutrition (ASPEN) recommended a simple method for predicting energy expenditure in critically ill obese patients, which is based on kcal per kg. No predictive formula has been shown to be superior in predicting calories of individual obese patients. Although IC remains the "gold standard" for measuring energy requirements, its use is limited by cost, availability of proper equipment, number of trained personnel, and the patient's respiratory status. In these circumstances, the predictive equations should be used as alternatives (Table 23.1).

Table 23.1 Predictive equations validated in critically ill obese patients

Authors	Equations
Harris and Benedict	Male: $66.5 + 13.8(\text{ABW}) + 5(\text{Ht}) - 6.8(\text{A})$
	Female: $655.1 + 9.6\ (\text{ABW}) + 1.8\ (\text{Ht}) - 4.7(\text{A})$
Mifflin and St. Jeor	Male: $10\ \text{W} + 6.26(\text{Ht}) - 5(\text{A}) + 5$
	Female: $10\ \text{W} + 6.26\ (\text{Ht}) - 5\ (\text{A}) - 161$
Ireton-Jones	Ventilator-dependent: $1784 - 11(\text{A}) + 5(\text{W}) + 244\ (\text{G}) + 239(\text{T}) + 804(\text{B})$
	Spontaneously breathing: $629 - 11\ (\text{A}) + 25\ (\text{W}) - 609\ (\text{O})$
SCCM/ASPEN*	Male and female: $11-14(\text{W})$

ABW, adjusted body weight; Ht, height (cm); A, age (years); W, actual weight (kg); G, gender (male=1, female=0); T, trauma; B, burn; O, obesity (if present=1, absent=0).
*Hypocaloric feeding equation.

Assessment and application of hypocaloric feeding

For critically ill obese patients, hypocaloric nutrition support is the recommended approach. Multiple studies have demonstrated improved metabolic control as well as outcomes in the ICU with this approach. Historically, hypocaloric feedings originated from the early use of the protein-sparing modified fast for the treatment of obesity in inpatient and outpatient settings starting in the early 1970s. This approach is in contrast to permissive under-feeding, which is also applied to lean critically ill patients. Permissive under-feeding reduces all macro- and micro-nutrition delivery, which leads to less energy, protein, carbohydrates, and other nutrients. On the other hand, hypocaloric feeding reduces the delivery of non-protein calories, which decreases total energy delivery without a reduction in protein and other micronutrients. Therefore lean body mass loss is minimized while allowing greater loss of fat mass. However, this should not be the primary objective for nutrition support during critical illness. The other rationale for the administration of hypocaloric feeding is to prevent the metabolic consequences of overfeeding, such as hypercapnea, fluid retention, and hypertriglyceridemia. High-protein hypocaloric feeding also can markedly improve insulin sensitivity and glycemic control.

For all classes of obesity where BMI is greater than 30 kg/m^2 and hypocaloric feeding is appropriate the goal caloric intake should not exceed 60–70% of energy requirements, calculated by IC or predictive equations. The weight-based formula from SCCM and ASPEN (11–14 kcal/kg) can be used alternatively. Appropriate protein delivery can promote protein synthesis and preserve lean body mass. Protein should be provided in a range of ≥ 2.0 g/kg ideal body weight per day for a BMI of 30–40 kg/m^2 patients and ≥2.5 g/kg ideal body weight per day for BMI > 40 kg/m^2 patients. It can be adjusted, if necessary, based on nitrogen balance measurements taken while monitoring the patients on feeding. Even in malnourished or depleted patients, a positive nitrogen balance can be achieved with hypocaloric intake (relative to energy expenditure) by increasing protein intake. The only possible contraindications to hypocaloric feeding would be progressive renal failure, hepatic encephalopathy, ketosis, or severe immune-compromised state.

Although hypocaloric feeding was initially designed for the parenteral route, enteral feeding is usually a preferred method for critically ill obese patients who have the ability to tolerate enteral feeding. Early enteral nutrition in the critically ill is thought to be beneficial through its effects on gut mucosal integrity and possible modulation of systemic immunity, the latter being particularly important for obese patients who already have a pre-existing inflammatory state.

Most standard as well as specialized feeding formulas will not satisfy 100% of protein requirements using a hypocaloric approach. There are newer "bariatric" or "immune-enhancing" formulas available that have a higher protein to calorie ratio. A useful option is to add protein modules to the standard formulas. Approximately 60–80% of the energy requirements should be provided through feeding formulas and the remainder should be fulfilled by extra protein substrates.

Obese patients are more likely to have increased abdominal pressure and risk of gastroesophageal reflux and aspiration. Delayed gastric emptying is also a common issue in obese patients because of their predisposition to clinical diabetes and its associated enteric neuropathy. For these reasons, selective feeding into the small bowel beyond the pylorus may be necessary to reduce the risk of gastroesophageal reflux and aspiration.

Pharmaconutrients

The use of certain pharmaconutrients in the critically ill is under active investigation in both obese and non-obese patients, with some positive outcomes reported particularly for the "immune-enhancing" formulas containing higher amounts of arginine and omega three fatty acids (N-3 FA).

Currently, N-3 FA (EPA and DHA) are used in critical care for improving antioxidant status and modulating immunity and inflammation. N-3 FA activate peroxisome proliferator-activated receptor (PPAR)–γ and PPAR-α, which increase insulin release and decrease inflammation by blocking macrophage migration into white adipose tissues and decreasing inflammatory cytokines. N-3 FA increases adiponectin levels and can reduce the incidence of non-alcoholic fatty liver changes in the obese population. Therefore, it is clear that N-3 FA may have some benefit for critically ill obese patients and a few studies support the effect of N-3 FA in severe obesity by decreasing systemic inflammation.

Arginine is a semi-essential amino acid that modulates vascular tone (vasodilatation) through nitric oxide synthase (NOS) pathways. Arginine reduces the effect of asymmetric dimethyl arginine (ADMA), which is a competitive NOS antagonist. Elevated levels of ADMA are found in chronic and acute disease states including obesity. In animal studies, arginine improved serum levels of glucose, triglycerides, long-chain fatty acids, and leptin and may even contribute to weight loss. Arginine increases hepatic blood flow and promotes wound healing. This may be particularly beneficial to critically ill obese patients who require surgical intervention or have severe injuries. Because arginine may be converted to nitric oxide contributing to hemodynamic instability, arginine should be used cautiously or may need to be avoided in patients with severe sepsis.

Many other potential pharmaconutrients and trace elements are under investigation for clinical use in critically ill obese patients. These agents include magnesium, zinc, leucine, glutamine, betaine, carnitine, citrulline, medium-chain triglycerides, and α-lipoic acid. Many of these agents have been shown to reduce the low-grade systemic inflammatory response syndrome (SIRS), improve insulin sensitivity, and preserve lean body mass. However, human data proving these effects is limited especially in the obese population and therefore standard use of these nutrients requires more studies to be performed.

Summary points

- The number of obese patients admitted to ICUs has increased as a result of the obesity epidemic.
- Nutritional assessment and support is a key element in proper management of critically ill obese patients. Estimating caloric requirements of critically ill obese patients with predictive equations is challenging as most of them were developed for the non-obese population. Currently, indirect calorimetry remains the gold standard for estimating energy requirements.
- Hypocaloric feeding is recommended for most critically ill obese patients. Hypocaloric feeding is intended to reduce non-protein calorie infusions, while maximizing protein sparing. The caloric goal should not exceed 60–70% of the energy requirement and a daily intake of at least 2.0–2.5 g/kg (ideal body weight) protein is required.
- This hypocaloric feeding regimen will prevent complications of overfeeding such as hyperglycemia and fluid retention while preserving lean body mass and promoting steady controlled weight loss.
- Further investigations are needed for clinical use of pharmaconutrients in critically ill obese patients, though some experimental studies have shown positive results.

Further reading

Hurt RT, Frazier TH, McClave SA, et al. Pharmaconutrition for the obese, critically ill patient. J Parenter Enteral Nutr 2011;35:60S–72S.

Kaafarani H, Shikora A. Nutritional support of the obese and critically ill obese patient. Surg Clin North Am 2011;91:837–855.

Kushner R, Drover J. Current strategies of critical care assessment and therapy of the obese patient (hypocaloric feeding): what are we doing and what do we need to do? J Parenter Enteral Nutr 2011;35:36S–43S.

Martindale RG, DeLegge M, McClave SA, et al. Nutrition delivery for obese ICU patients: delivery issues, lack of guidelines, and missed opportunities. J Parenter Enteral Nutr 2011;35:80S–87S.

Martino JL, Stapleton RD, Wang M, et al. Extreme obesity and outcomes in critically ill patients. Chest 2011;140:1198–1206.

McClave SA, Martindale RG, Vanek VW, et al. Guidelines for the Provision and Assessment of Nutrition Support Therapy in the Adult Critically Ill Patient: Society of Critical Care Medicine (SCCM) and American Society for Parenteral and Enteral Nutrition (A.S. P.E.N.). J Parenter Enteral Nutr 2009;33:277–316.

McClave SA, Kushner R, Van Way CW, et al. Nutrition therapy of the severely obese, critically ill patient: summation of conclusions and recommendations. J Parenter Enteral Nutr 2011;35:88S–96S.

Palghi A, Reed JL, Greenburg I, et al. Multidisciplinary treatment of obesity with a protein-sparing modified fast: results in 668 outpatients. Am J Public Health 1985;75:1190–1194.

Paolini JB, Mancini J, Genestal M, et al. Predictive value of abdominal obesity vs. body mass index for determining risk of intensive care unit mortality. Crit Care Med 2010;38:1308–1314.

Port AM, Apovian C. Metabolic support of the obese intensive care unit patient: a current perspective. Curr Opin Clin Nutr Metab Care 2010;13:184–191.

Index

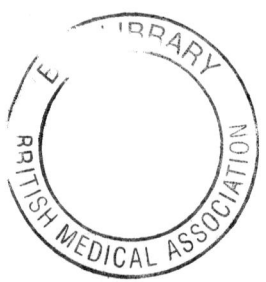